Home Care for the Client Needing Rehabilitation

Home Care for the Client Needing Rehabilitation

Jetta Lee Fuzy, RN, MS
Director of Development and Training
Health Education, Incorporated
Fort Lauderdale, Florida

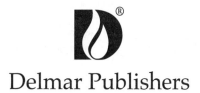

Delmar Publishers

an International Thomson Publishing company I(T)P®

Albany • Bonn • Boston • Cincinnati • Detroit • London • Madrid
Melbourne • Mexico City • New York • Pacific Grove • Paris • San Francisco
Singapore • Tokyo • Toronto • Washington

NOTICE TO THE READER

Cover Design by Brian J. Sullivan, Essinger Design Associates

Delmar Staff

Publisher: Susan Simpfenderfer
Acquisitions Editor: Dawn Gerrain
Developmental Editor: Debra Flis
Project Editor: Elizabeth A. LaManna
Production Manager: Wendy A Troeger
Team Assistant: Sandra Bruce

Art and Design Coordinator: Vincent S. Berger
Production Coordinator: John Mickelbank
Marketing Manager: Katherine Hans
Marketing Coordinator: Glenna Stanfield
Editorial Assistant: Donna L. Leto

COPYRIGHT © 1999
By Delmar Publishers
a division of International Thomson Publishing Inc.
The ITP logo is a trademark under license.

Printed in the United States of America

For more information, contact:
Delmar Publishers
3 Columbia Circle, Box 15015
Albany, New York 12212-5015

International Thomson Publishing Europe
168–173 Berkshire House
High Holborn
London, WC1V7AA
England

Nelson ITP, Australia
102 Dodds Street
South Melbourne,
Victoria, 3205 Australia

Nelson Canada
1120 Birchmount Road
Scarborough, Ontario
M1K5G4, Canada

International Thomson Publishing France
Tour Maine-Montparnasse
33 Abenue du Maine
75755 Paris Cedex 15, France

International Thomson Editores
Seneca 53
Colonia Polanco
11560 Mexico D. F. Mexico

International Thomson Publishing GmbH
Königswinterer Strasse 418
53227 Bonn
Germany

International Thomson Publishing Asia
60 Albert Street
#15–01 Albert Complex
Singapore 189969

International Thomson Publishing—Japan
Hirakawa-cho Kyowa Building, 3F
2-2-1 Hirakawa-cho, Chiyoda-ku,
Tokyo 102, Japan

ITP Spain/Paraninfo
Calle Magallanes, 25
28015-Madric, Expana

1 2 3 4 5 6 7 8 9 10 XXX 03 02 01 00 99 98

Library of Congress Cataloging-in-Publication Data
Fuzy, Jetta Lee.
    Care of the rehabilitation client / Jetta Lee Fuzy.
        p.   cm.
    Includes Index.
    ISBN: 0-8273-7931-5
        1. Medical rehabilitation. 2. Home care services. 3. Home nursing. 4. Rehabilitation nursing. I. Title.
        [DNLM: 1. Rehabilitation Nursing--methods. 2. Rehabilitation--methods. 3. Home health Aides.   WY 150.5 F996c 1998]
    RM930.F89 1998
    610.73--dc21
    DNLM/DLC
    for Library of Congress   97-45220
                                      CIP

A service of I⟮T⟯P®

Table of Contents

Preface

As the home care aide (HCA) takes on more and more responsibility in home care, this expanding role includes participation in the rehabilitation process of home care clients. It is important for the HCA to understand rehabilitation, the common conditions frequently seen in the home requiring rehabilitation, the equipment used, and the HCA's role in returning the client to the highest possible level of function.

This specialty training program has been designed to provide HCAs with training over and above their basic education and to give HCAs the necessary training to prepare them to take care of these clients in a knowledgeable and supportive manner.

Chapter 1 is a review of those body systems commonly involved in caring for clients in a rehabilitation program. Common disorders in each of these systems are reviewed in Chapter 2. Skilled therapies play an important role in the rehabilitation process and are the focus of Chapter 3. Various types of equipment often used in rehabilitation are discussed in Chapter 4 including adaptive equipment, safety equipment, personal care equipment, exercise equipment, and supportive devices. Chapters 5 and 6 focus on specially trained HCAs and the specific care they are expected to provide their clients including treatments and procedures.

Pain reduction and control is briefly reviewed in Chapter 7. Client and family education and the HCA's role is discussed in Chapter 8. Safety and emergency procedures, abuse issues, and psychosocial influences are the focus of the last three chapters.

As more clients are discharged from rehabilitation centers and hospitals to the home environment, home care aides as assistants to the skilled nurse will be expected to play an active part as a member of the rehabilitation team.

The specially trained HCA must understand the importance of caring for the client as a whole person, not just the body part that is weakened or impaired. The psychosocial, multicultural, and holistic aspects of each client must be considered in the care plan. Because many members of the home care team play a part, the HCA has to be trained to understand each team member's role and function as the client progresses through the rehabilitation process and into self-care.

In addition, the clients themselves and their families play an important role in the rehabilitation process, and the HCA, as the client's advocate, can be influential in motivating and encouraging their valuable participation.

Whether providing the client with assistance in activities of daily living, ambulation, or exercise, the HCA with advanced training in rehabilitation will no doubt spend valuable and skillful periods of time in the home.

ACKNOWLEDGMENTS

The author wishes to thank Jeleen Fuzy for her valuable input regarding both the structure and content of this training manual. Without her patience and encouragement, I could not have completed this project.

The author and Delmar wish to thank the following individuals for reviewing the manuscript and providing valuable comments:

Judith Bradley, RN
Director of Rehabilitation Services
Alacare Home Health Care Services
Irondale, Alabama

Diana Hendon, RN, CRRN
Alacare Home Health Care Services
Irondale, Alabama

Joann Jeannenot, AA
Director, Home Care Department
Hampshire County VNA
Northampton, Massachusetts

Michelle Livesay, RN, BSN
Inservice Coordinator
Total Home Health Care
Lubbock, Texas

Linda Mitchell, RN, BS
Visiting Nurse Association
Denver, Colorado

Eunice Warner, RN
Director of Home Health
Rogue Valley Manor Home Health Care
Medford, Oregon

Introduction

The HCA who works as a rehabilitation specialist plays a vital role in home care today. He or she will become a great asset to the agency he or she works for and to the clients cared for with this newly acquired knowledge.

The client in a rehabilitation progam will experience great adjustments and losses and the HCA's ability to assist him or her emotionally and physically will be very rewarding. The HCA will be involved with other health care professionals who have dedicated their lives to assisting disabled persons toward a new life. The opportunity to work with disabled clients brings health caregivers self-fulfillment as they greatly impact these person's recoveries.

Returning the client to self-care is a long-term goal in all home health care situations. This is especially true of clients in a rehabilitation program who have lost the ability to care for themselves in many areas. How much self-care rehbilitation is possible depends on the client and the degree of injury involved. There is a big difference between returning the client with arthritis to self-care and that of a survivor of a brain injury. However, the main goal is for the health care team to determine the optimal level of self-care that can be obtained and then strive to meet that level, whatever it might be. Because every human being has the need to feel useful, caring for oneself must include some functions that the person considers useful.

Minimal self-care could be simply performing the activities of daily living for oneself such as feeding and bathing. At the other extreme, self-care could involve helping a client who has had a stroke learn to drive a car again. Many clients who have had strokes go home from the hosptal to lead normal lives through the rehabilitation process. Independence is a major factor and independence may mean simply performing ADLs or being back in the workplace and collecting a paycheck on a regular basis. The health care team must all agree onthe plan and the goals and discuss them with the client and family on an on-going basis. The client with a chronic disease that causes increasing disabilities needs to be kept at a realistic level of rehabilitation during the course of the illness. For example, the client with Multiple Sclerosis (MS) will have long periods of remission where the symptoms will not be as severe. During these periods, the patient will feel more useful but must be cautioned not to overdo activities and create fatigue. This may also be true of other chronic disabilities.

Self-care deficits are common in clients suffering from MS, arthritis, Parkinson's disaease, stroke, brain and spinal cord injuries, vision impairments, and emotioal illnesses. Any of these clients may experience physical, emotional, and perceptual deficits. It is up to the physician and the therapist to determie if these deficits are permanent or temporary and what measures should be taken to restore the client to an optimal level of function in view of the limitations.

The return to self-care must involve the physical, psychological, socioeconomic, spiritual, and environmental elements. The therapist and all the members of the health care team that have been previously discussed must consider all five areas before a comprehensive self-care plan can be considered successful.

There are always gonig to be new treatments and devices to assist the client. It is the specially trained HCA's responsibilty to keep abreast of these in the future. Remember these clients are not handicapped because that means a social disadvantage for an individual. These clients are disabled in that they have a limitation in their activity because of an injury of illness. With the specially trained staff, the client may change his or her disability into ability through the process of restoration to a heathy conditionand a useful capacity through the rehabilitation process.

The key element to any rehabilitation process is hope. The client must have hope that the program will eventually improve his or her quality of life; hope that tomorrow will be a day to look forward to because he or she will be a more active, independent, and healthy person.

List of Client Care Procedures

Anatomy and Physiology

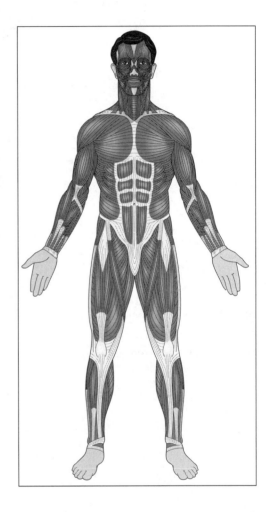

OBJECTIVES

Upon reading this chapter and completing the review questions, the home care aide should be able to:

1. Describe the musculoskeletal system and the various injuries that can occur to muscles and bones.

2. Recognize and describe the organs included in the urinary and gastrointestinal systems and understand the process of liquid and solid waste elimination from the body.

3. Understand the nervous system and the function of the brain and spinal cord.

KEY TERMS

atrophy

contracture

elimination

involuntary muscles

voluntary muscles

INTRODUCTION

To prepare HCAs to become rehabilitation specialists, it is important that they review the four body systems and the common disorders of each that is usually seen in home situations where rehabilitation is prescribed. These body systems are the musculoskeletal system, the urinary system, the gastrointestinal system, and the nervous system. A basic understanding of anatomy and physiology enables the HCA to understand the body and how it works.

THE MUSCULOSKELETAL SYSTEM

The musculoskeletal system is the system most often affected by disorders requiring rehabilitation. Motion of the body is made possible by the muscular system. The musculoskeletal system provides the framework upon which the body moves. In addition, it protects the body and gives it form. The three main parts of the musculoskeletal system are:

1. *Muscles*—Groups of muscles work together to perform a body motion. This is accomplished by the contraction of one group and the relaxation of an opposite group of muscles. If a muscle is not used for a long period of time, it tends to shrink, or **atrophy**. A **contracture**, or a permanent shortening of a muscle, can occur and limit the client's ability to move easily.

atrophy muscle decreasing in size

contracture when muscle tissue becomes drawn together or shortened because of spasm or paralysis (can be permanent or temporary

2. *Bones*—There are 206 bones in the skeletal system and they are moved by muscles. There are four types of bones: long bones, such as the femur (thigh bone); short bones, such as the phalanges (finger bones); irregular bones, such as the vertebrae (spinal column); and flat bones, such as those comprising the rib cage. Normal bones are hard and unbending and are made up of living cells. The center is filled with marrow, a soft "filling" where blood cells are produced. At the place where one bone connects to another, there is always a joint which allows movement. Joints such as the shoulder, hip, and knee are encased in a capsule along with a fluid called synovial fluid which cushions the joint. Injuries to joints (which include injuries to ligaments or tendons) are called sprains. A break or a crack in a bone is called a fracture.

3. *Connective Tissue*—Connective tissue includes:
   a. Ligaments—Ligaments are white fibers which connect bone to bone and support the joint.
   b. Tendons—Tendons connect muscles to bones.
   c. Cartilage—Cartilage cushions joints.

Connective tissue plays a major role in movement. Without the ligaments, tendons, and cartilage, the body would have no mobility.

voluntary muscles the movement of the body controlled by the conscious brain

involuntary muscles muscles that receive messages from the nervous system but work automatically without the person being aware of it

Helpful Hints: When caring for a client with muscle and/or bone pain or weakness, the HCA must discuss the care plan with the supervisor. This ensures that each client receives the care appropriate to the illness.

Skeletal muscles are **voluntary muscles** because movement is controlled by the conscious brain. Figures 1–1A and 1–1B show the skeletal muscles. **Involuntary muscles** receive messages from the nervous system and work automatically without a person's awareness. Examples of involuntary muscles are the walls of most organs such as the heart.

It is important for the HCA to be familiar with the most prominent bones of the skeleton so that when caring for clients needing rehabilitation, he or she will understand how the muscles, bones, and connective tissues work, particularly when they are injured.

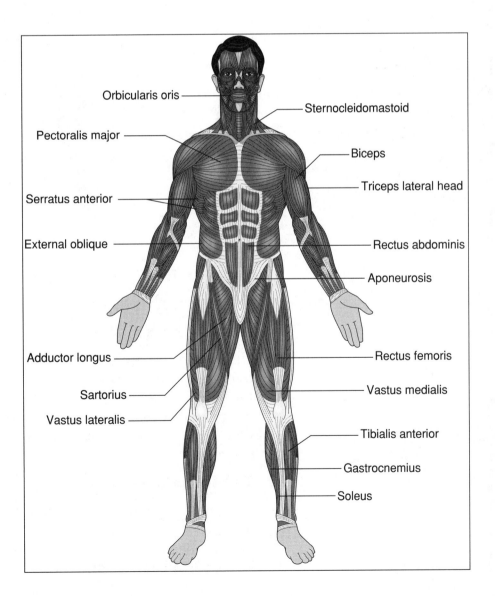

Figure 1–1A Anterior view of the muscular system

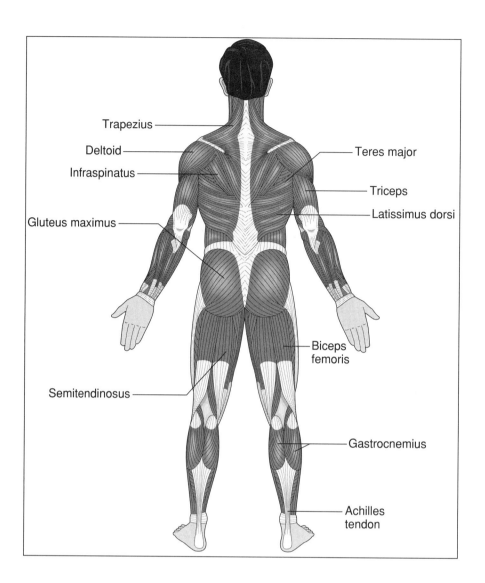

Figure 1–1B Posterior view of the muscular system

Figure 1–2 shows the most prominent bones in the adult human skeleton.

THE URINARY AND GASTROINTESTINAL SYSTEMS

The urinary system and the gastrointestinal (GI) system are important in the rehabilitation process because bowel and bladder training are often included in restoring the client to optimal function. The following description of the anatomy and physiology of these two systems is limited to those areas involved in waste elimination.

The Urinary System

The urinary system is responsible for eliminating waste products through urine. These waste products, which result from burning food for energy, are taken from the blood. The process of urinating is called **elimination**. The urinary system is composed of the

elimination the process of urinating

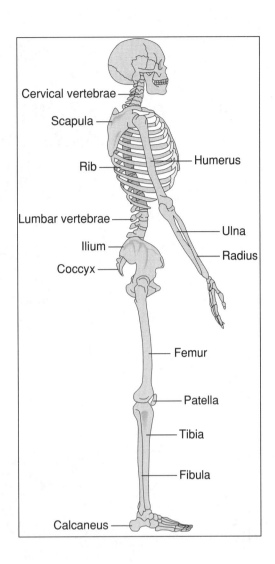

Figure 1–2 Adult human skeleton

kidneys, ureters (the tubes leading from the kidneys to the bladder), the urinary bladder, and the urethra (the tube leading from the bladder to the outside of the body). Figure 1–3 shows the urinary system.

The Gastrointestinal System

Elimination also includes waste matter from the bowels through the gastrointestinal system. The GI system breaks food down so it can be absorbed in the bloodstream and taken to the body cells to be used for nutrition and energy. The gastrointestinal system begins at the mouth and includes the mouth, pharynx, esophagus, stomach, small intestine, large intestine, and anus, where it ends. Figure 1–4 shows the digestive system.

Elimination occurs when the waste matter in the rectum (which is the lower eight to ten inches of the colon or large intestine) is expelled through the anus (which is the body opening from the rectum).

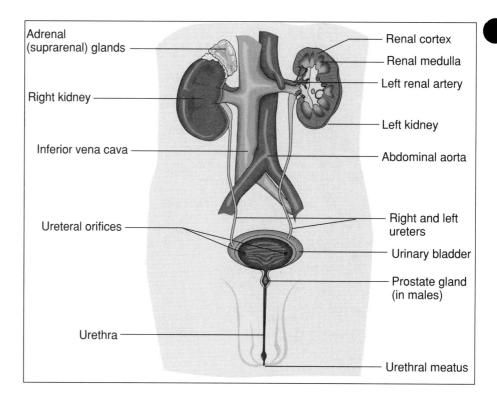

Figure 1–3 The urinary system

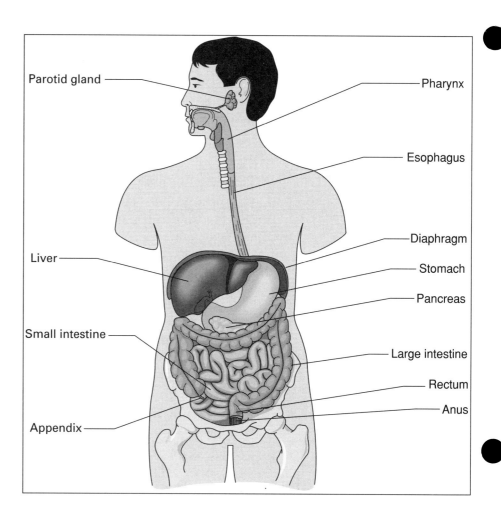

Figure 1–4 The digestive system

THE NERVOUS SYSTEM

The nervous system controls the activities of the body and is comprised of two main parts: the central nervous system (the brain and the spinal cord) and the peripheral nervous system (the cranial nerves and spinal nerves). The sensory organs—eyes, ears, nose, taste buds, and skin—are usually considered part of the nervous system.

The nervous system consists of nerve endings throughout all parts of the body and is made up of cells called neurons. Neurons transmit messages through tissues including nerve fibers and muscles. Nerve cells are like electrical wires and have an insulating cover called the myelin sheath. When nerve cells are injured in the brain and spinal cord, they do not repair themselves and it is necessary for another part of the brain to take over the function of the damaged area. The rehabilitation process is necessary to help clients relearn activities after such injury or damage has occurred.

The brain is the most important organ of the body because it controls every action and reaction a person experiences. The brain is protected by bones (the cranium) and a cushion of fluid which surrounds the spinal cord. Figures 1–5A and 1–5B show the brain and skull, respectively.

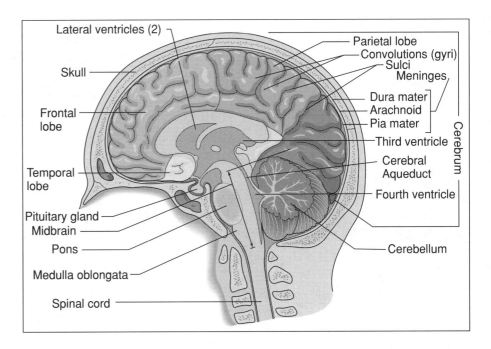

Figure 1–5A Cross section of the brain

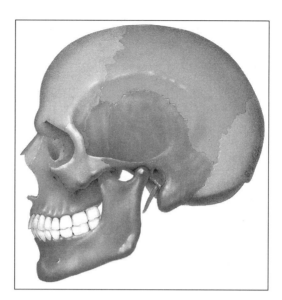

Figure 1–5B Lateral view of the skull

The brain has five main parts:

1. *Cerebrum*—The cerebrum is divided into the left and right hemispheres. The right hemisphere controls the activity of the left side of the body and the left hemisphere controls the activity of the right side of the body. Some of these functions include thinking, memory, emotions, and reasoning.

2. *Cerebellum*—The cerebellum coordinates muscular activity and balance.

3. *Pons*—The pons is the base of the brain and controls involuntary function in numerous organs including the heart, lungs, stomach, and intestines.

4. *Medulla*—The medulla is the pathway from the brain to the spinal cord and controls involuntary function with the pons. Some of these functions include heartbeat, breathing, and digestion.

5. *Spinal Cord*—The spinal cord contains twelve pairs of cranial nerves and thirty-two pairs of spinal nerves which branch to all parts of the body. The nerves act as the highways through which the messages from the brain travel to the various parts of the body. Figure 1–6 shows the central and peripheral nervous system.

It is important for the HCA to understand the brain and spinal cord function to better understand the body's reaction to injuries in these important organs.

As common disorders are discussed, the musculoskeletal, urinary, gastrointestinal, and nervous systems will be referred to repeatedly because they play a major role in the rehabilitation process.

Helpful Hints: It is important for the HCA to discuss with the supervisor where brain and spinal injuries have occurred in the client. This enables the HCA to understand the client's particular illness and his or her response to the care provided.

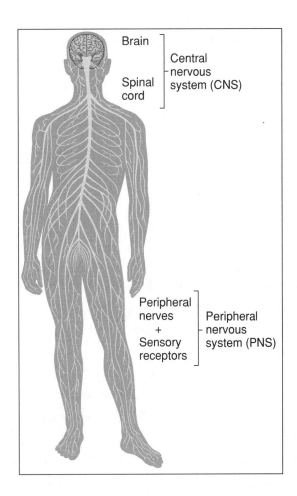

Figure 1–6 Central and peripheral nervous system

REVIEW QUESTIONS

1. The three main parts of the musculoskeletal system that provide function and structure are
   _____ , _____ , and _____ , _____ .
2. There are _____ bones in the skeletal system.
3. The four types of bones are: _____ , _____ , _____ ,
   and _____ .
4. Which of the following is not an example of an involuntary action?
   a. breathing
   b. heartbeat
   c. standing up
   d. blinking your eyes
5. Which of the following is the most important organ in the human body?
   a. the heart
   b. the liver
   c. the brain
   d. the nose

6. Which of the following is included in the GI system?
   a. bladder
   b. brain
   c. large intestine
   d. muscles
7. Which of the following is not considered a connective tissue?
   a. ligaments
   b. tendons
   c. cerebellum
   d. cartilage
8. True or False? The spinal cord is part of the nervous system.
9. True or False? Involuntary muscles can be found on the walls of most organs.
10. True or False? If a muscle is not used for a long period of time it tends to atrophy.
11. True or False? The urinary system is responsible for eliminating waste products taken from the blood resulting from burning food for energy.

Match the system in the left column to its function in the right column:

12. _____ nervous system   a. eliminates waste products
13. _____ urinary system   b. breaks down food
14. _____ gastrointestinal system   c. includes eyes, ears, and skin
15. _____ musculoskeletal system   d. protects the organs and body
16. Unscramble the following key term from the chapter: nttcruacroe _____

CHAPTER 2

Common Disorders in Which Rehabilitation is Indicated

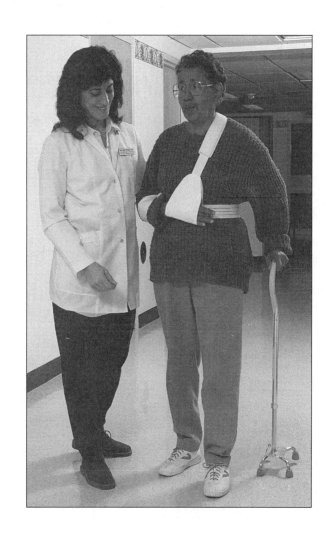

OBJECTIVES

Upon reading this chapter and completing the review questions, the home care aide should be able to:

1. Describe common disorders in which rehabilitation is indicated.

2. Describe the treatments involved for common disorders requiring rehabilitation.

3. Recognize common disorders associated with the systems of the body and the home care aide's role in each.

4. Be familiar with complications that may arise when taking care of clients requiring rehabilitation.

KEY TERMS

activities of daily living (ADL)
aphasia
arteriosclerosis
arthritis
cerebral vascular accident (CVA)
hypertension

incontinence
paraplegic
quadraplegic
range of motion (ROM)
spasms

INTRODUCTION

This chapter focuses on common disorders seen in clients who require rehabilitation. It is important that the HCA understand these diseases and how they affect the client's well being.

THE MUSCULOSKELETAL SYSTEM

The musculoskeletal system is the system most often affected by injuries or illnesses that require rehabilitation. The HCA specializing in caring for clients undergoing rehabilitation should be familiar with these common illnesses and injuries.

Arthritis

arthritis   an inflammation of the joint causing pain and limitation of movement of the joint

Arthritis is an inflammation of a joint which causes pain and limitation of movement in the joint. Sometimes these joints swell. There is no cure for arthritis. Arthritis is usually defined as two types: rheumatoid arthritis and osteoarthritis.

Rheumatoid arthritis is a chronic inflammatory disease which causes damage to cartilage and bone. It usually occurs in women between the ages of forty and sixty. Symptoms occur because of damage to the lining of the joints and include fatigue, weakness, general aches, stiffness, pain, and limited movement. Morning stiffness is the greatest obstacle to overcome in rehabilitation. Figures 2–1A, B, C, and D show deformities as a result of rheumatoid arthritis.

The treatment for rheumatoid arthritis is exercise, aspirin, and anti-inflammatory drugs. Occasionally, surgery may be necessary to replace joints. Physical therapy (PT) and rehabilitation are focused on controlling pain and increasing strength, motion, and function.

Osteoarthritis is the most common disease of the joints. It is different from rheumatoid arthritis in that the surface of the cartilage is changed. Pain usually occurs after use of the joint and is relieved by rest. The joints usually involved in osteoarthritis are the fingers, shoulders, knees, hips, and spine.

Treatments for osteoarthritis are aspirin, anti-inflammatory drugs, and pain medicine. Occasionally, the joint will be injected with cortisone. Surgery, including joint replacement, is some-

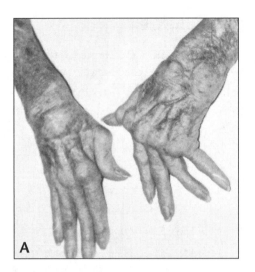

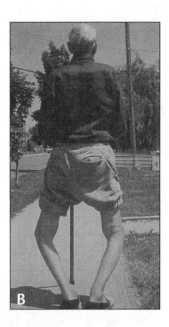

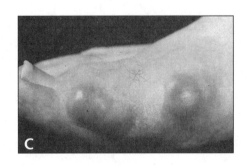

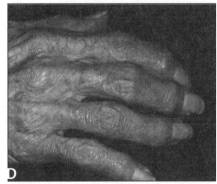

Figure 2–1 Joint deformities resulting from rheumatoid arthritis

activities of daily living (ADLs)
tasks performed each day such as toileting, bathing, dressing, feeding, grooming, homemaking, and other activities

range of motion (ROM) exercises which move each muscle and joint through a full range of motion to assist the patient in an exercise program

Helpful Hints: If the client's discomfort increases from one visit to the next, the supervisor should be notified. Perhaps the client should take pain medications before ambulating or another problem related to exercises might be present about which the therapist should know.

times the choice of treatment. This is very successful with larger joints such as the hip. PT is usually ordered to improve function through exercise and an increase in the **activities of daily living (ADLs). Range of motion (ROM)** exercises also are important to increase flexibility to maintain joint mobility.

Arthritis is one of the most common musculoskeletal disorders seen in the home care situation (often occurring along with other illnesses). When the HCA participates in an exercise program following the plan of care with the client who has arthritis, he or she should encourage the client to move the body even when pain and stiffness are present. An occupational therapist (OT) may be involved in making the home safe for the client with arthritis.

Osteoporosis

Osteoporosis is defined as reduced amounts of normal bone tissue which causes softening of the bone. The bones become brittle and, therefore, are easily fractured. Calcium levels are reduced in the bones, leaving the bone weak. Osteoporosis is more common in women and is thought to be caused by a lack of hormones following menopause. Osteoporosis is thought to be worsened by lack of mobility. Complications include the following:

- Vertebrae may collapse causing curvature of the spine
- Fractures occur easily
- Hip fractures are common from falls and cause serious nursing problems (to be discussed in more detail in Chapter 7).

Figure 2–2 shows the disease process, treatments, and special care techniques for osteoarthritis, rheumatoid arthritis, and osteoporosis.

Condition	Disease Process	Treatment	Special Care
Osteoarthritis	Breakdown (degeneration) of joints, such as ankles, knees, and hips are most commonly involved. Movement is painful and condition is progressive.	Medication to relieve pain; physiotherapy to maintain mobility; light massage and heat; ambulatory aids to reduce pressure in joints; weight reduction; surgery in selected cases.	Give positive, emotional support; carry out heat treatments, massage, and ROM exercises, as ordered.
Osteoporosis	Defective bone formation and maintenance. Bones become brittle and are easily broken. Complications: fractures, kidney stones, and loss of height and posture. More common in females than males.	Keep resident as active as possible; diet adequate in protein and vitamins C and D, and calcium; maintain adequate fluid intake; hormone therapy.	Encourage food and fluid intake. Assist in exercise. Report pain; apply support as needed. Emotional support must not be overlooked.
Rheumatoid Arthritis	Inflamation of joint lining (synovium). Joint changes cause painful muscle spasms, flexion, and deformities. Signs and symptoms may temporarily disappear (remission). Flare-ups may be related to emotional stress.	Drugs to reduce pain and inflammation; heat treatments for comfort; exercise when inflamation subsides; surgery in selected cases.	Provide emotional support. Provide self-help devices such as long shoe horns and grab bars. Carry out heat treatments and ROM exercises, as ordered.

Figure 2–2 Common orthopedic problems in the elderly

Fractures

Fractures are breaks or cracks in a bone. There are five types of fractures:

1. A simple or closed fracture—the bone is broken but not in pieces and does not break through the skin.
2. A compound or open fracture—the bone breaks through the skin.
3. A comminuted fracture—the bone breaks into many pieces.
4. A greenstick fracture—the bone has a simple crack which does not penetrate the bone completely.
5. An impacted fracture—one bone fragment is forced into another bone or bone fragment.

Figure 2–3 shows four of the five types of fractures, excluding an impacted fracture.

Broken bones heal slowly because bone cells reproduce slowly. Hardening of the bone relies on calcium deposits. Resistance to infection in the bone is poor because blood supply is poor. Signs of a fracture include:

- pain
- swelling
- bruising
- limited movement
- bleeding and color change in the skin at the fracture site.
- shock
- a grating sound produced during movement
- distortion of normal body alignment; deformity

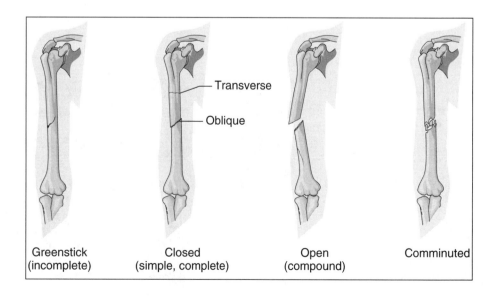

| Greenstick (incomplete) | Closed (simple, complete) | Open (compound) | Comminuted |

Figure 2–3 Types of fractures

- loss of function
- numbness
- loss of rigidity

In the geriatric client, the most common fractures are hip, shoulder, and vertebrae. In order for fractures to heal, the bone must be kept in proper alignment and immobile. Treatment for a fracture is often the use of a cast or a splint. Some fractures are treated with traction in which the broken ends of the bone are pulled into alignment. With skin traction, a belt or strap is used and weights are attached to ropes. With skeletal traction, a metal pin is placed through the bone and alignment is maintained with weights.

Contractures

A contracture is a permanent tightening or shortening of a muscle. It is usually caused from inactivity and can often be prevented. Contractures cannot be reversed and often worsen once they start. Once the client has a contracture, three serious nursing problems occur: limited movement, difficulty with positioning, and poor hygiene. Symptoms of a contracture are stiff joints or joints that do not move at all because the muscle shortens, freezing the joint. Figure 2–4 shows a client with a contracture.

There are other disorders of the musculoskeletal system, but they do not usually play a role in home care rehabilitation. These include bursitis, sprains, strains, dislocations, contusions, surgical amputation, tendonitis, cancer of the bone, and muscular dystrophy.

Helpful Hints: In elderly clients, bones heal slowly and the HCA must encourage the person to be patient and follow the physician's orders carefully.

Helpful Hints: The best HCA care is reflected in preventing complications such as contractures by methods of positioning, exercise, or ambulation, as ordered.

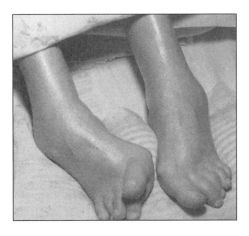

Figure 2–4   Contractures are a complicaton of inactivity

THE URINARY AND GASTROINTESTINAL SYSTEMS

The urinary system and the gastrointestinal systems play important roles in the rehabilitation process because the client who requires rehabilitation often requires bowel and bladder retraining because of incontinence.

Incontinence

incontinence the inability to control bladder or bowel function

The most commonly seen disorder requiring rehabilitation associated with the urinary and gastrointestinal systems is incontinence of the bladder or bowel. **Incontinence** is defined as the inability to control bladder or bowel function. Incontinence can occur at any age; however, the elderly are more susceptible for the following reasons:

- neurological damage, such as a stroke
- poor muscle control
- medications
- infections of the urinary tract
- lack of awareness
- arteriosclerosis that affects the blood vessels supplying the bladder
- inability to get to the bathroom in time
- fecal impactions
- misuse of laxatives and enemas earlier in life

Urinary incontinence may be short term and handled with the use of disposable undergarments (see Figure 2–5). However, it can be chronic and serious enough to require a retention catheter.

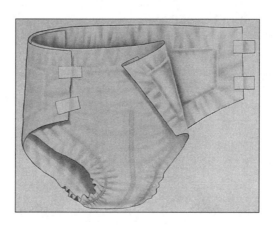

Figure 2–5 A disposable brief

Bowel incontinence is caused by nerve damage, weakened muscles, and occasionally by fecal impactions. The treatment for bowel incontinence is bowel training exercises and a retraining process. The HCA plays an important role in this retraining process. (The HCA's role will be discussed in greater detail in Chapter 5.) Retraining has proven successful in rehabilitation for both bowel and bladder incontinence. Figure 2-6 shows the "ABCs" of incontinence.

Incontinence is not a normal part of aging and causes many physical and psychological problems. It is very embarrassing for both the client and the family. Incontinence can be prevented if bowel and bladder management programs are started early enough. These programs can restore self-care and self-respect to the client and prevent serious complications associated with incontinence.

Clients who are incontinent have greater risk for complications including:

- skin breakdown
- bladder infections
- fecal impactions
- poor wound healing
- pressure ulcers
- poor infection control

Incontinence impacts the musculoskeletal system, the urinary and gastrointestinal systems, and the nervous system. It is important, therefore, for the HCA to understand the cause, treatment, and role they play in preventing and controlling this serious disorder.

THE NERVOUS SYSTEM

Disorders of the nervous system can result in the client's inability to speak, hear, see, touch, and think. They can affect the person's mobility and, as already stated, his or her bowel and bladder functions.

Parkinson's Disease

Parkinson's disease is a chronic illness in which transmission of messages in the brain are disrupted, causing problems in balance and walking. Speech may also be affected because of the client's inability to move facial muscles. The symptoms include:

- mask-like facial expression
- trembling
- stooped posture

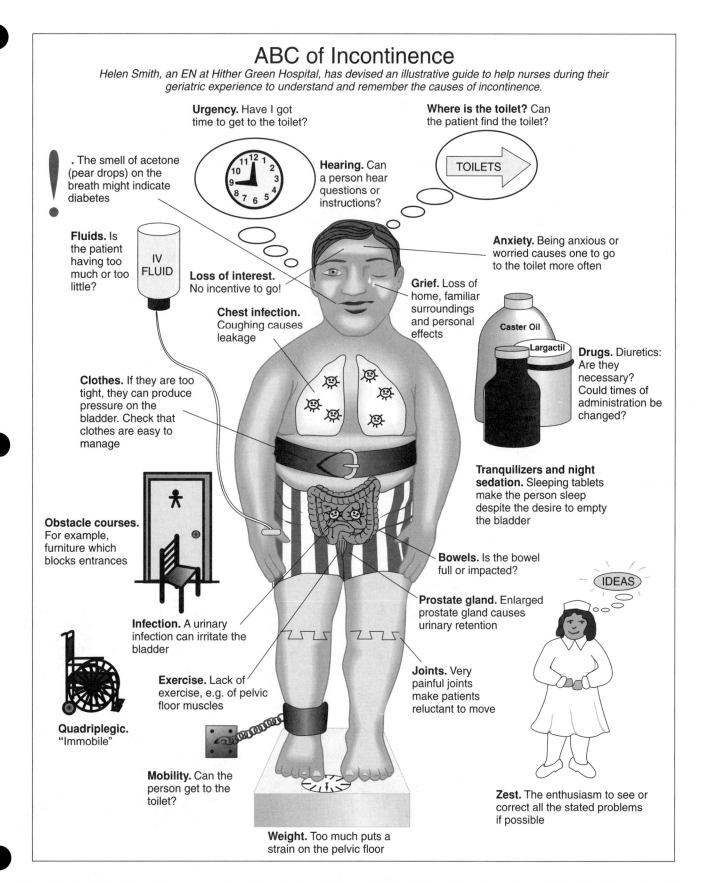

Figure 2–6 ABC of incontinence reproduced by kind permission of *Nursing Times* where it was first published on November 13, 1985.

- stiff muscles
- slow walking movements (a shuffle)
- slurred speech
- drooling

Figures 2–7A and B show a client with Parkinson's disease.

Mental awareness is not usually affected and depression is a common response. Clients with Parkinson's disease have rigid muscles that cause them to fall and they are injured more frequently than other clients. Incontinence is a common problem as well as contractures. Rehabilitation, therefore, especially as a preventative measure, is important. There are medications that control some of the symptoms. Clients with Parkinson's disease deteriorate into severely disabled patients. Clients in the latter stages are frequently seen in nursing homes, but in the early stages, are commonly seen in home health situations and require physical therapy (PT), occupational therapy (OT), and speech therapy (ST).

Brain and Spinal Injuries

Brain and spinal injuries cause complex nursing problems and frequently result in paralysis. A **paraplegic** is a client whose lower body is paralyzed and a **quadriplegic** is a client whose four extremities are paralyzed. Figure 2–8 shows a client who is a quadriplegic.

> **Helpful Hints:** Changes in gait, speech, or mental status must be reported immediately because they might be signs that action should be taken quickly to prevent further impairment.

paraplegic a client whose lower part of the body is paralyzed

quadriplegic a client in whom all four extremities are paralyzed

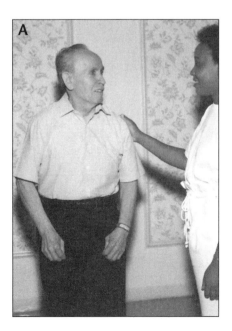 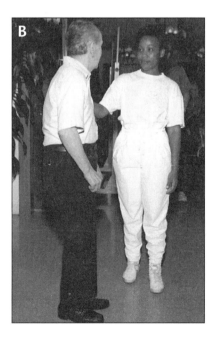

Figure 2–7 The typical posture, from a ventral and lateral view, of a client with Parkinson's disease.

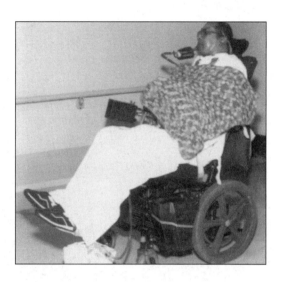

Figure 2–8 This client is a quadriplegic and needs assistance with activities of daily living.

The disabilities depend on the location of the injury and/or disease involved. The following functions can be impaired:

- judgment and decisions
- body functions
- memory and recall
- sensation
- thought processes

Injury or diseases to the brain stem can cause:

- impaired respiration
- impaired heart rate and rhythm
- abnormal blood vessel size
- abnormal internal organ functioning

Diseases and injuries of the autonomic nervous system (part of the peripheral nervous system) affect the sense organs and cause impairment in touch, temperature, pain, vision, hearing, taste, equilibrium, and smell. Some associated disorders include cataracts, glaucoma, and diabetic retinopathy caused by small vessel deterioration in the retina. Rehabilitation is important for the paralyzed client in order to maintain the highest possible quality of life.

Multiple Sclerosis

Multiple Sclerosis (MS) is a loss of the covering that insulates the nerves which cause them to lose their function. It begins in young adulthood with visual problems, weakness, and fatigue and progresses to blindness, contractures, paralysis, incontinence, and respiratory problems. The care plan should focus on the prevention of complications such as:

- contractures
- incontinence

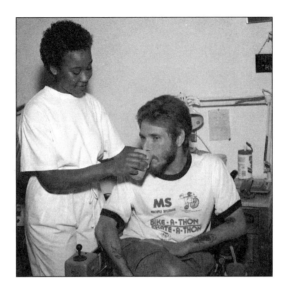

Figure 2–9 An aide provides care for a client with MS.

cerebral vascular accident (CVA; also called a stroke) a disorder in which blood flow to parts of the brain are blocked caused by a hemorrhage, a thrombus, an embolus, or arteriosclerosis

hypertension high blood pressure

arteriosclerosis a build-up of cholesterol in the arteries

Helpful Hints: TIA episodes might occur during the night and should be reported immediately if the client appears to have slight changes in speech or weakness. The HCA should take vital signs and call the supervisor, thereby allowing a physician time to prescribe treatment which could prevent a stroke.

- decubitus ulcers
- poor mobility
- depression

Rehabilitation is a major factor in the lives of these clients (see Figure 2–9) and the HCA may be caring for clients with MS at home along with PTs, OTs, STs, respiratory therapists (RTs), and medical social workers.

Cerebral Vascular Accident (CVA)

A **cerebral vascular accident** (**CVA**), also called a stroke, is a disorder in which blood flow to parts of the brain is blocked. It can be caused by a hemorrhage, a thrombus, an embolus, or arteriosclerosis. CVAs are the third leading cause of death in the United States and are characterized by the following risk factors:

- **hypertension**—high blood pressure
- **arteriosclerosis**—a build-up of cholesterol in the arteries
- transient ischemic attack (TIA)—a reduced blood supply to the brain which causes the client to black out.
- smoking
- immobility
- obesity

A TIA is not actually a stroke but is instead a warning. It may last a few minutes to many hours.

The signs and symptoms of a stroke depend on which part of the brain is affected and the amount of damage that occurs to the brain (see Figure 2–10). Damage might be permanent or blood vessels around the area could create a new blood supply. If

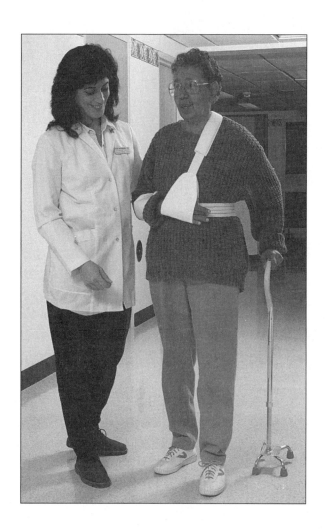

Figure 2–10 This client had a stroke, resulting in paralysis of the right side of her body.

aphasia loss of language or speech

the left side of the brain is damaged, paralysis will occur on the right side of the body along with **aphasia**, the inability to speak. The client will show signs of anxiety and perform slowly. If the right side of the brain is affected, paralysis will be on the left side of the body. The client will have problems with perception which will interfere with ADLs. This client becomes quick and impulsive.

Symptoms that can occur with either left or right side brain damage include:

- sensation loss in the affected extremities
- inability to use the paralyzed side of the body
- impaired vision
- emotional instability
- a drooping of the eyelid and the muscles on one side of the face
- **spasms** in the paralyzed limbs

spasm an involuntary movement of muscle

The client who has had a stroke is at risk for the following complications:

- increased risk of contractures
- pressure sores (decubitus ulcers)
- pneumonia
- constipation
- blood clots
- incontinence

Caring for a client who has had a stroke is one of the greatest challenges in home health care today. It requires a team of health care personnel including the home care aide. There are four major goals in the rehabilitation program for a client who has had a stroke:

1. maintain the self-care level that the client has remaining
2. prevent complications
3. rehabilitate the client in ADLs, bowel and bladder training, exercise and activities, and communication
4. maintain the client's highest level of emotional and psychological health.

Recovery from a stroke is a slow rehabilitative process in which even the smallest success should be considered significant. It is important to encourage the client to do as much for himself or herself as possible. Complications can be prevented through proper positioning, range of motion exercises, good nutrition and fluid balance, bowel and bladder training program, and increasing the client's communication skills with patience and concern

The rehabilitation program is long and complex. A comprehensive care plan with realistic goals is important. The recovery time and degree of rehabilitation is different for each client and the amount of permanent disability varies. The client, however, can return to some levels of self-care and independence with careful and supportive assistance. The HCA must remain patient, concerned, and helpful while teaching and encouraging the client at all times. The HCA must never show signs of impatience with the client or family members during the healing process.

Helpful Hints: Motivating the client who is recovering from a stroke is an HCA function. A positive attitude and praise are essential.

REVIEW QUESTIONS

1. Define the two types of arthritis:
   a. Rheumatoid Arthritis
   b. Osteoarthritis

2. In the geriatric patient, the most common fractures are _____ , _____ , and _____ .

3. List the four goals of rehabilitating a patient who has had a stroke.

    a.

    b.

    c.

    d.

4. Which of the following is a reason why the elderly are more susceptible to incontinence than other groups of patients?

    a. poor muscle control

    b. poor eyesight

    c. poor skin elasticity

    d. poor hygiene

5. Which of the following is a complication associated with clients who are incontinent?

    a. poor balance

    b. confusion

    c. pressure ulcers

    d. fatigue

6. In sprain and spinal injuries, which of the following functions is not impaired?

    a. sensation

    b. thinking

    c. digestion

    d. respiration

7. Symptoms that occur in a client who has had a CVA do not include:

    a. impaired vision

    b. chest pain

    c. poor sensation

    d. confusion

8. True or False? A contracture is a temporary tightening of a muscle.

9. True or False? Bowel incontinence is caused by nerve damage and weakened muscles.

10. True or False? If the left side of the brain is damaged by a stroke, paralysis will occur on the left side.

11. True or False? A TIA is not actually a stroke.

Match the item in the left column to its definition in the right column:

12. _____ paraplegia   a. tightening of the muscle

13. _____ quadriplegia   b. paralysis of lower body

14. _____ arthritis   c. inflammation of joint

15. _____ contracture   d. paralysis of all four extremities

16. Unscramble the following key term from the chapter: ctnicneennio _____

CHAPTER 3

Multiple Disciplines

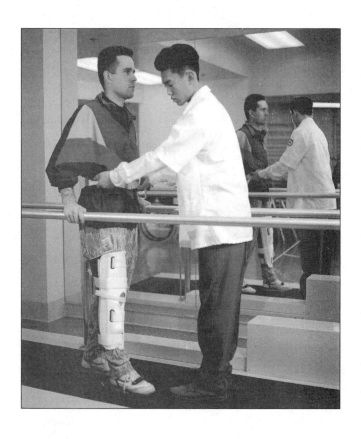

OBJECTIVES

Upon reading this chapter and completing the review questions, the home care aide should be able to:

1. Understand the HCA and PT care plans and their role in each.
2. Recognize the multidiscipline members of the team and each one's role and function in the rehabilitation process.
3. Be familiar with the goals and treatment regimens of PT.

KEY TERMS

care plan

medical social worker (MSW)

multidiscipline

occupation

occupational therapist (OT)

physical therapist (PT)

PT plan of care

rehabilitation centers

respiratory therapist (RT)

speech therapist (ST)

INTRODUCTION

multidiscipline the group of various therapies (disciplines) on the rehabilitation team

The term **multidiscipline** is frequently used in rehabilitation and refers to the different therapists (disciplines) included in the rehabilitation team. These include the physical therapist, speech therapist, occupational therapist, respiratory therapist, and medical social worker.

PHYSICAL THERAPY

physical therapist (PT) uses exercises and treatments to increase mobility

The **physical therapist (PT)** is a health care professional who uses exercises and other treatments to help clients increase mobility. Figure 3–1 shows a physical therapist helping the client increase mobility.

The physical therapist is responsible for evaluating and treating clients with musculoskeletal and neuromuscular problems because of disease, injury, or developmental disabilities. In home care cases, the physical therapist is usually required to assess and evaluate the client, consult with the physician in developing a treatment plan, design a physical therapy care plan that other members of the team can utilize, and initiate and monitor the physical therapy treatments.

Helpful Hints: The HCA may be supervised by the PT when there is no nurse on the case. PTs are considered "skilled therapists," recognized by insurance companies as the case manager for clients in a rehabilitation program.

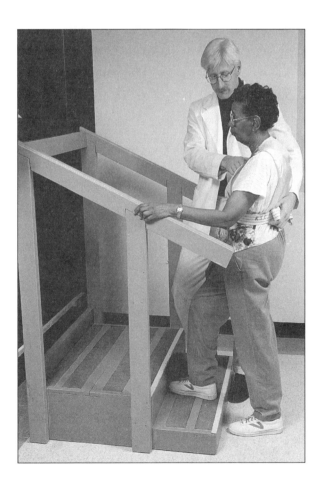

Figure 3–1 The physical therapist teaches the client how to use her body again and become strong after an accident or surgery.

There are physical therapy assistants who frequently make home visits after the rehabilitation plan is initiated. Some of the treatment procedures physical therapists use include those which:

- increase strength, endurance, coordination, and range of motion
- stimulate motor activity to improve activities of daily living
- teach the use of assistive devices
- attempt to relieve pain through prescribed therapy

rehabilitation centers outpatient PT where large equipment is needed

The physical therapist begins a program in the hospital that continues after discharge and in the home. Some clients receive some of their PT as outpatients in **rehabilitation centers** where large pieces of equipment are involved. These include parallel bars for support when learning to walk, whirlpools, kitchen and bathroom set-ups for wheelchair teaching, and large exercise equipment for strengthening bones and muscles. Figure 3–2 shows a PT working with the client on the parallel bars at a rehabilitation center. Equipment in the home is usually smaller. Sometimes, clients need a period of both outpatient and in-home therapy until they graduate to in-home therapy only.

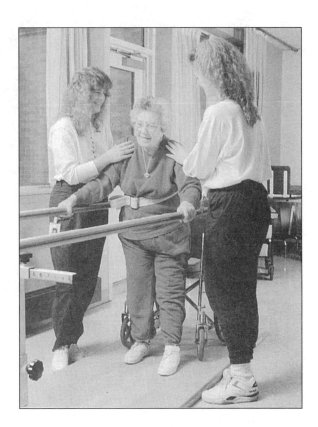

Figure 3–2 Rehabilitation centers have large pieces of equipment such as parallel bars for support.

The goals of physical therapy in the rehabilitation process involve the following:

1. Improve the quality of life for this client by returning him or her to the maximum level of function.
2. Increase the client's productivity.
3. Offer a safe environment in the home with lowered risk of injury.
4. Decrease pain.
5. Decrease medications, particularly those prescribed for pain.
6. Promote self-care and independence.
7. Increase strength, flexibility, and endurance in light of the present disability.
8. Increase self-esteem and emotional wellness.
9. Increase day-to-day activities, both at work and leisure.
10. Increase the client/caregiver's confidence for discharge.

Figure 3–3 shows a physical therapist helping the client to improve his ability to walk.

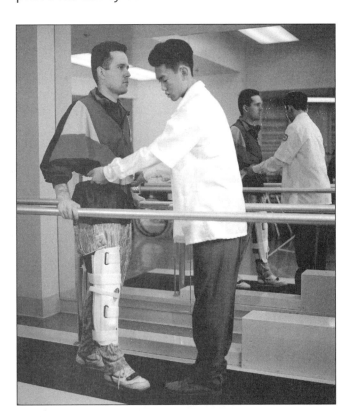

Figure 3–3 The physical therapist works with the client to improve mobility.

Some of the treatments in which the client might be involved are:

- therapeutic exercises
- transfer training
- gait training

- ultrasound
- electrotherapy
- prosthetic training
- muscle strengthening and flexibility exercises
- pain management
- traction
- massage

PT plan of care care plan specific to PT care and treatments

The physical therapist develops a **PT plan of care** which should be reviewed by other members of the care team including the HCA. The plan of care contains important information such as:

- client's diagnosis (onset or injury)
- level of function or functional limitations
- home environment appropriateness to rehabilitation
- equipment necessary
- problems
- client goals
- anticipated rehabilitation potential
- discharge plans
- discharge date
- client's emotional and mental status
- role of other team members, including the family, client, nurse, and HCA

"Therapists in home care cannot function in isolation. They must interact with nursing supervisors, staff nurses, and aides to coordinate care plans and ease integration of their services into the agency . . . Changing perspectives demand that the whole team—client, physician, and all caregivers—develop the therapy program holistically" (Hirn and Boin, p.11–12).

OCCUPATIONAL THERAPY

occupational therapist (OT) assists in restoring muscle coordination and strength by increasing the client's activity and independence

The **occupational therapist (OT)** is a health care professional who provides rehabilitative services to persons with physical injuries, psychosocial problems, or developmental disabilities. Figure 3–4 shows an occupational therapist helping a client apply a splint. The occupational therapist helps clients restore muscle coordination and strength, assists with increasing activities, and helps the client become more independent. The OT teaches the client to take part in his or her day-to-day care with such activities as personal care, eating, dressing, recreation, homemaking activities, and grooming. It is the OT's responsibility to establish a plan and monitor the plan for the activities of daily living. A care-

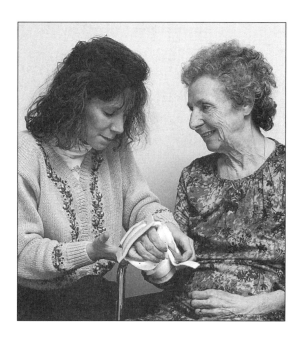

Figure 3–4 The occupational therapist applies a splint to the client's right arm.

care plan the written plan for daily care and treatments for the client that all disciplines follow

Helpful Hints: In some cases, a PT or an OT assistant may visit the client. The HCA serves as the eyes and ears of the therapist and the nurse.

occupation how the client is occupied in day-to-day living activities

Helpful Hints: In home care, the HCA might be supervised by an OT rather than the PT or the nurse if there is no other professional on the case.

speech therapist (ST) assists to improve speech and communication abilities

ful evaluation must be done and the OT and the PT usually work closely together to accomplish goals. A **care plan** for OT is also important and the OT should include the HCA in assisting the client through the exercises documented in his or her care plan. This is especially true in the area of setting goals and encouraging the client to participate in meeting the goals. In addition, the OT is instrumental in adapting the home to the client's disability.

The difference between OT and PT is that occupational therapy applies all of the above treatments or procedures to help clients regain their "occupation." **Occupation** refers not only to a person's work, but also to how they are occupied in day-to-day living activities that include leisure and play activities. For example, Mrs. Sandra Brown had a stroke with a severe disability and weakness in her left leg and arm which caused functional limitations in walking. The physical therapist was ordered by the physician to teach Mrs. Brown to walk again. The occupational therapist was ordered by the physician to teach Mrs. Brown techniques of self-care such as dressing, preparing meals, bathing, and caring for herself and her home. The two worked together to restore Mrs. Brown to the highest possible level of function. The level achieved might not be the normal level of function, but it will be the best that could be attained with the limitations involved.

SPEECH THERAPY

The **speech therapist (ST)** is a health care professional who assists the client to improve speech and communication. Clients who have a loss of speech have many psychological problems associated with difficulty in communication. The speech therapist sets up a long-term program to reteach clients to speak after strokes and other disabilities. This is a very slow and painful process for both the client and the family, and the HCA, as a member of the team, can be helpful in reinforcing the speech therapist's care plan. The speech therapist provides exercises and directions in the home for the family and other caregivers to incorporate into the daily plan. It is often the HCA's responsibility to oversee these exercises. In addition, the ST evaluates the swallowing ability of the client to determine if special feeding and/or drinking techniques are necessary to keep the patient's nutrition at the highest possible level. In some cases, a registered dietitian may be consulted for special diet orders.

Helpful Hints: Changes in speech, especially deteriorations, should be reported because they might be signs of a disease process.

RESPIRATORY THERAPY

respiratory therapist (RT) restores the best level of breathing through breathing exercises

The **respiratory therapist (RT)** is a specialist who restores the best possible level of breathing during rehabilitation. This includes having the client perform breathing exercises to increase lung capacity. As with any of the care plans, the caregiver or the HCA must reinforce the exercises in order to enhance the rehabilitation process.

MEDICAL SOCIAL WORKER

medical social worker (MSW) deals with spiritual, economic, and psychosocial problems

A **medical social worker (MSW)** is a person who deals with the spiritual, economic, community resource, and psychosocial problems of the client during the rehabilitative process. Good communication between the MSW and the other members of the multidisciplinary team is vital to the success of the program. Depression is a common response to disabilities and can affect both the client's and family's acceptance of that disability. The MSW assesses the psychosocial affects of the rehabilitation program and suggests actions to be taken to improve the situation.

Figure 3–5 shows a medical social worker comforting a client.

Helpful Hints: HCAs spend more time in the home than any other member of the health care team. Therefore, they may be an important source of input concerning the client's mental attitude toward the plan of care and whether or not the services of a social worker are needed.

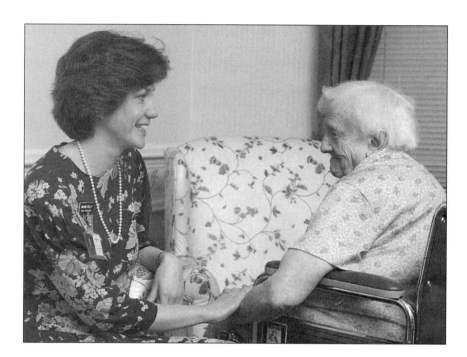

Figure 3–5 The social worker is concerned with the client's psychosocial needs.

REVIEW QUESTIONS

Match the functions with the person who performs it in the rehabilitation process:

1. _____ Reteaches daily activities   a. PT
2. _____ Assesses mobility levels   b. OT
3. _____ Restores breathing   c. RT
4. _____ Reteaches speaking and communication d. MSW
5. _____ Assists with psychosocial problems e. ST
6. Tell what goal the PT is working toward for the following clients.

   a. Mrs. Peggy Zimmerman had a stroke. Her rehabilitation process has been delayed because of depression.

      Goal:

   b. Mr. Steven Brown has severe arthritis and has been increasing his pain medication to dangerous levels.

      Goal:

   c. Mrs. Sally Lowry's daughter is concerned that her mother will fall in the shower.

      Goal:

   d. Mr. Dean Peterman, after hip surgery, cannot ambulate to the bathroom as yet.

      Goal:

7. Indicate with a "yes" or "no" what would *not* be included in the PT plan of care in the following list:

    a. _____ client goals

    b. _____ functional level

    c. _____ allergies

    d. _____ diet

    e. _____ emotional status

    f. _____ discharge plan

    g. _____ client's diagnosis

8. Unscramble the following key term from the chapter: niedicitsliupml _____

Rehabilitation Equipment

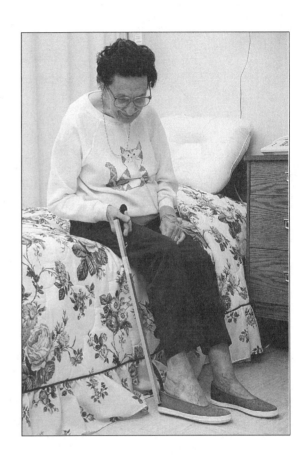

OBJECTIVES

Upon reading this chapter and completing the review questions, the home care aide should be able to:

1. Recognize and describe adaptive equipment and their uses.
2. Recognize and describe personal care devices and their uses.
3. Recognize and describe safety devices and their uses.
4. Recognize and describe supportive devices and their uses.
5. Recognize and describe exercise equipment and their uses.

KEY TERMS

adaptive equipment	rehabilitation equipment
exercise equipment	safety devices
personal care devices	supportive devices

INTRODUCTION

rehabilitation equipment
helps the client recover or
improve activity

Equipment that helps clients recover or improve activity when a disability occurs is called **rehabilitation equipment**. Assistive devices are the most common pieces of equipment used in rehabilitation cases. There are five types of assistive devices:

1. adaptive equipment
2. personal care devices
3. safety devices
4. supportive devices
5. exercise equipment

ADAPTIVE EQUIPMENT

adaptive equipment   assists the
client with ADLs

Devices designed to assist disabled clients with their activities of daily living include **adaptive equipment**. Each item is modified by the designer to allow clients to perform activities they otherwise could not do. Some adaptive devices are:

- aerosol can adapter with a trigger to help the client hold down the spray
- plates with high edges
- cutlery with built-up handles
- feeding cups with nonspill tops
- angled cutlery for people with limited arm motion
- long-handled tools for taking things from high shelves
- lowered tables and counters for wheelchair-bound clients
- one-handed knife
- food guards for plates to keep food from spilling out
- hand clips for people who cannot grip handles

    Figure 4–1 shows a client using adaptive equipment.
    Figure 4–2 shows adaptive equipment designed to help clients feed themselves.

PERSONAL CARE DEVICES

personal care devices   special
equipment designed to encourage self-care

It is important that the client in rehabilitation do as much for himself or herself as possible. This is especially true of personal care, and special equipment has been designed just for this purpose. The following is a list of some **personal care devices**:

- long-handled brush and comb
- long-handled sponge for bathing
- nail care equipment adapted for one hand use
- grooming aids with built-up handles for easier grooming
- shoe grabbers and shoehorns with long handles

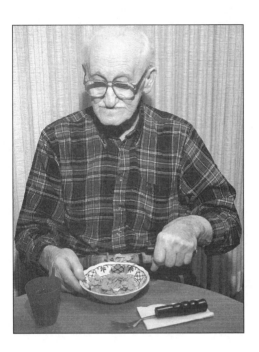

Figure 4–1 The client feeds himself using a special cup and a foam-handled fork and spoon.

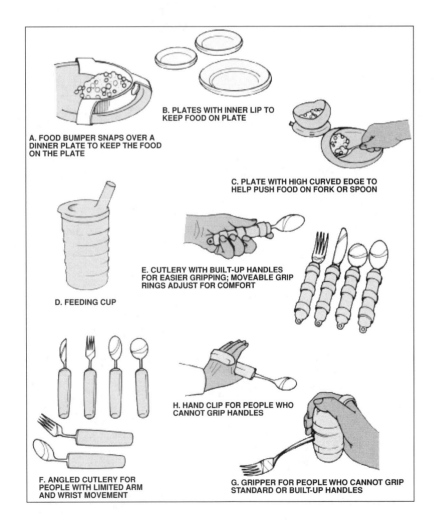

Figure 4–2 Special devices assist the elderly and handicapped to feed themselves.

- dressing stick
- zipper aid
- stocking aid to help clients pull up stockings
- button loop
- trouser aid

Figures 4–3 and 4–4 show some examples of personal care devices.

Helpful Hints: Sometimes it is faster for the HCA to perform the personal care activities than to allow the client to perform these activities themselves. Remember, however, that the goal is always for the client to reach the highest level of self-care possible.

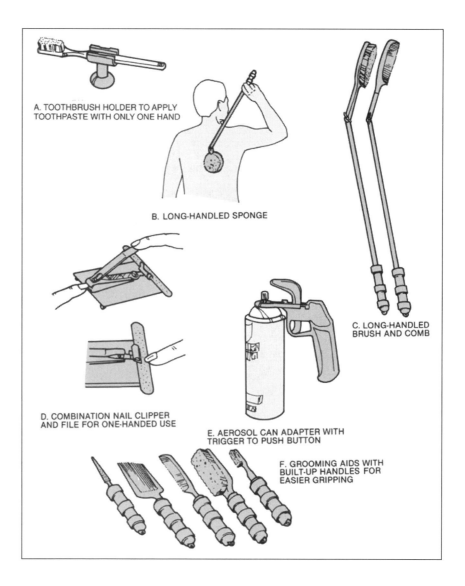

A. TOOTHBRUSH HOLDER TO APPLY TOOTHPASTE WITH ONLY ONE HAND

B. LONG-HANDLED SPONGE

C. LONG-HANDLED BRUSH AND COMB

D. COMBINATION NAIL CLIPPER AND FILE FOR ONE-HANDED USE

E. AEROSOL CAN ADAPTER WITH TRIGGER TO PUSH BUTTON

F. GROOMING AIDS WITH BUILT-UP HANDLES FOR EASIER GRIPPING

Figure 4   Personal care devices

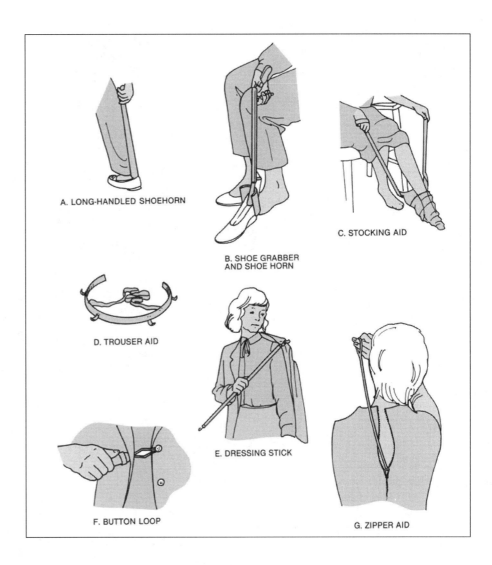

A. LONG-HANDLED SHOEHORN

B. SHOE GRABBER AND SHOE HORN

C. STOCKING AID

D. TROUSER AID

E. DRESSING STICK

F. BUTTON LOOP

G. ZIPPER AID

Figure 4–4 Adaptive devices for grooming and bathing

safety devices equipment used to lower the risk of client injury

Helpful Hints: If the HCA observes an unsafe environment or a situation that could be improved by installing safety devices, he or she should discuss this with the supervisor, the nurse, or the PT on the case.

SAFETY DEVICES

Because of the high risk of injury for clients who are unstable and have limited mobility, safety devices are an important part of the home setup during rehabilitation. The following is a list of some **safety devices** used in the home:

- Locking wheels and side rails for beds, as well as client call buttons.
- Devices such as whistles, bells, and intercoms so that clients are able to call for help any time they are unassisted or alone.
- Locking guards for the wheels of wheelchairs for safe transfer (see Figure 4–5).
- Guard rails along corridor walls for assistance in walking.
- Strong banisters and extra rails along steps and stairways.
- Supportive rails in bathrooms for tubs, showers, and around commodes.
- Ramps to assist clients get in and out of the home.

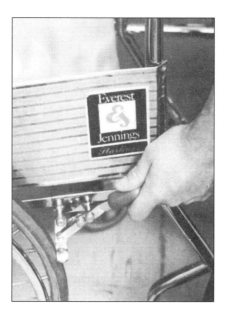

Figure 4–5 Always lock the wheels of the wheelchair before transferring a client to the chair.

- Gait belts to support clients when ambulating.
- Raised toilet seats (see Figure 4–6).
- Bath and shower seats (see Figure 4–7).

SUPPORTIVE DEVICES

supportive devices protect the client from falling when ambulating

Supportive devices are used to protect the client from falling when ambulating. The following is a list of some supportive devices:

- canes (quad canes, blind canes, and seat canes)
- walkers
- crutches

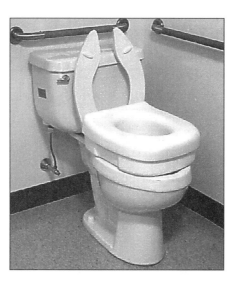

Figure 4–6 Raised portable toilet seats allow the client easier transfer on to and off of the toilet.

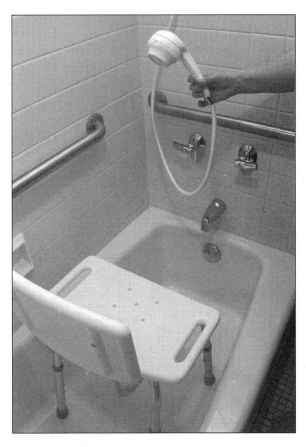

Figure 4–7 Bath chairs are often used to assist the client to get in and out of the bathtub safely.

Helpful Hints: The HCA must be familiar with safety and supportive devices in order to use them correctly and to act as a role model for the client and family.

- gait belts
- Hemi-walkers
- seat walkers
- wheeled walkers
- wheelchairs and the numerous accessories available.
- antitip wheelchairs

Figures 4–8, 4–9, and 4–10 show some of the supportive devices used by home care clients.

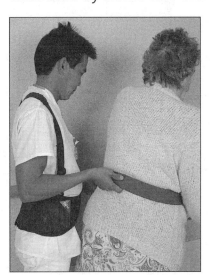

Figure 4–8 A gait belt is often used to ambulate a client who is unsteady on his or her feet. If the client starts to fall, the aide can safely ease the client to the floor by holding onto the gait belt.

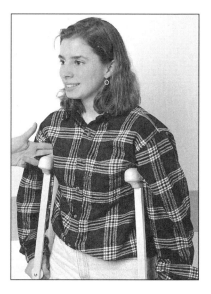

Figure 4–10 Crutches are fitted to the client by ensuring there is a width of two fingers between the top of the crutch and the client's armpit.

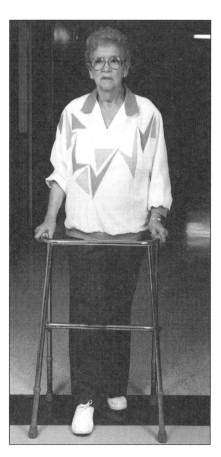

Figure 4–9 The client lifts the walker, places it in front of himself or herself, then steps forward.

EXERCISE EQUIPMENT

Exercise is usually ordered by the physician and planned by the physical therapist or occupational therapist. The HCA should be familiar with the equipment used because he or she might have to assist the client with the exercises prescribed. The following is a list of some **exercise equipment** used during rehabilitation:

- pulley devices for arm and back strengthening exercises
- Thera-bands (stretchable rubber strips to strengthen upper arms)
- stationary bicycles for strengthening legs
- physioballs for hand-to-eye coordination
- exercise putty for strengthening hands
- weights to strengthen legs and hands during ambulation

The devices listed above are only a sample of the available equipment used in rehabilitation. The more complex equipment is ordered by a physician, the physical therapist, or the occupational therapist.

exercise equipment equipment to improve the strength and mobility of the client

Helpful Hints: If there is a piece of equipment in the home with which the HCA is not familiar, he or she should ask the supervisor for a demonstration of how it is used.

Helpful Hints: The HCA should never assist the client with exercises unless the therapist and/or nurse have included them on the HCA Care Plan.

All equipment companies have excellent client education materials available for guiding the family and the client, as well as the HCA, in the proper use of their equipment. The safe use of all equipment can be assured at a case conference with all of the caregivers present.

REVIEW QUESTIONS

1. A one-handed knife is an example of _____ _____.
2. Bath and shower seats are examples of _____ _____.
3. An example of exercise equipment is _____.
4. Which of the following is *not* an example of assistive devices?
   a. pulley devices
   b. wheelchair
   c. overhead lighting
   d. dressing stick
5. A long-handled sponge for bathing is an example of:
   a. exercise equipment
   b. supportive devices
   c. personal care devices
   d. adaptive equipment
6. True or False? All assistive devices are considered adaptive equipment.
7. True or False? The HCA should be familiar with assistive devices in order to help the client use them properly.
8. Unscramble the following key term from the chapter: xreesiec nitqepeum _____

CHAPTER 5

HCA Roles and Functions

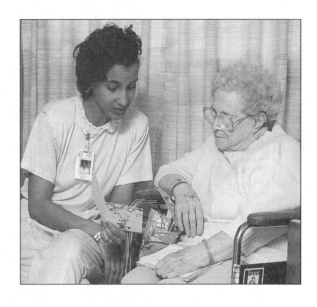

OBJECTIVES

Upon reading this chapter and completing the review questions, the home care aide should be able to:

1. Understand case conferences and the role of the HCA.

2. Define client goals and expected outcomes, including problems.

3. Understand the aspects and importance of communication and documentation.

4. Describe the general rules basic to all documentation.

5. Recognize additional areas of concern for clients requiring rehabilitation.

KEY TERMS

case conferences	nursing care plan
documentation	payors of home care
expected outcomes	signs
goals	symptoms
HCA care plan	

INTRODUCTION

As the HCA is given more responsibility through specialization, the nurse and the HCA will become a close working team. The two important aspects involved in this team are communication and coordination.

The HCA's roles and functions will increase and become more specific to caring for the client with unique needs, such as one who requires rehabilitation. Some of the new roles and functions for HCAs caring for the client requiring rehabilitation are:

- Having a knowledge of the common disorders associated with rehabilitation and the treatments involved.
- Providing personal care to the client requiring rehabilitation by assisting with bathing and dressing, and at the same time, encouraging the client to do as much as possible to return to the highest level of self-care.
- Providing management of the home to make it a clean and safe environment in which the client can recuperate.
- Using principles of good body mechanics to conserve energy and prevent injury for both the HCA and the client.
- Understanding the principles of rehabilitation to reinforce PT, OT, and ST programs.
- Using proper transfer and ambulation techniques to safely increase mobility and strength in the client.
- Providing psychosocial support to the client and family.
- Understanding the skilled nurse's role and observing and reporting changes in the client's progress to the supervisor.
- Participating in case conferences.
- Offering procedures such as range of motion exercises, positioning, and so forth, to assist the client in recuperation.

CASE CONFERENCES

case conference   meetings of all members of the health care team to analyze the client's case

Meetings that are held periodically with all members of the health care team to analyze the management of the client's case and to point out problem areas and possible changes in the care plan are called **case conferences**. Figure 5–1 shows members of the health care team meeting for a case conference. In rehabilitation cases, case conferences should be held every two to four weeks. It is important that all the disciplines involved in the case receive input and that documentation is accurate on the case conference form. The HCA on the case should be included in the conference and the HCA care plan updated at this time.

The specially trained HCA who participates in rehabilitation case conferences can provide important information to the other members of the team. Figure 5–2 shows the communication process between the HCA and other members of the health care team. The members involved in rehabilitation case conferencing

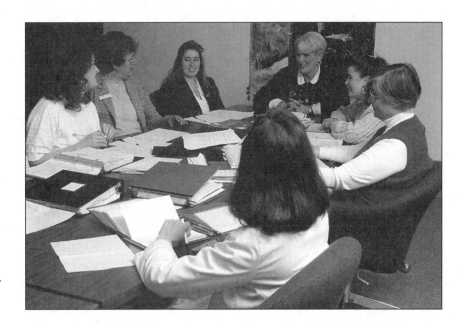

Figure 5–1 Case conferences are attended by the members of the interdisciplinary team.

Helpful Hints: There are times when the HCA's input will make a great difference in the success of the case conference.

might include the physician, the physical therapist, the occupational therapist, the speech therapist, the dietitian, the medical social worker, the skilled nurse, and the home care aide. Sometimes case conferencing is done over the telephone in case conference calls. It is the responsibility of all health care workers to keep up to date on the results of case conferences. If the HCA misses a conference, it is still his or her responsibility to obtain the updated information from the nurse or supervisor.

The case conference includes discussion in the following important areas:

1. common team goals
2. team member's individual care plans and treatment plans
3. problems and problem-solving
4. client status by means of an evaluation process

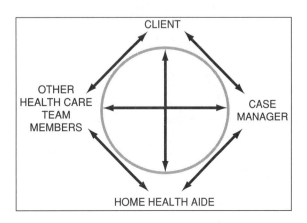

Figure 5–2 The HCA interacts with all members of the health care team.

goals purposes or objectives to work toward

5. new orders to the care plan
6. client **goals** and outcomes, and the progress being made toward them.

All case conferences should be documented in terms of measurable outcomes for the client. Usually, the skilled nurse is the case manager and, therefore, is responsible for the documentation and communication to other members of the team. The HCA should prepare for case conferences carefully and professionally as an important member of the management team.

As the team prepares the client for discharge, it becomes more and more important that case conferences be held and goals assessed.

nursing care plan plan the nurse follows which consists of problems (nursing diagnoses) and the long- and short-term goals to meet those problems

HCA care plan plan the HCA follows which is created by the nurse and updated every two weeks

CLIENT GOALS AND OUTCOMES

When the nurse in charge of the case of a client requiring rehabilitation determines the appropriate nursing diagnoses (nursing problems) for that client, those become the basis for the **nursing care plan** and the **HCA care plan**. Figure 5–3 shows a client care plan. At the same time, the nurse defines the client's long-term

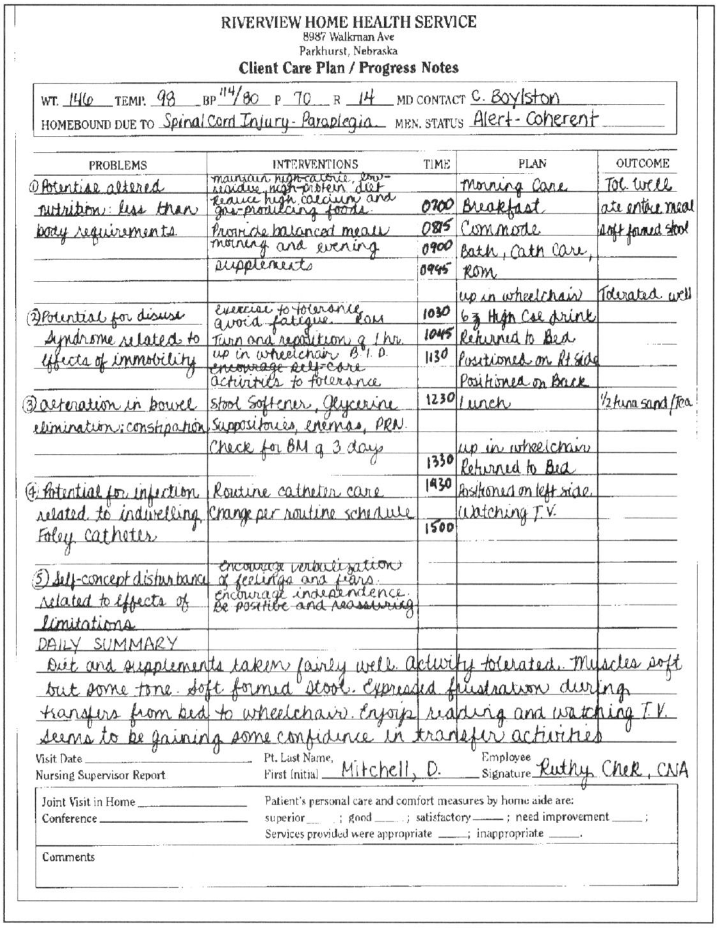
RIVERVIEW HOME HEALTH SERVICE
8987 Walkman Ave
Parkhurst, Nebraska
Client Care Plan / Progress Notes

WT. 146 TEMP. 98 BP 114/80 P 70 R 14 MD CONTACT C. Boylston
HOMEBOUND DUE TO Spinal Cord Injury - Paraplegia MEN. STATUS Alert - Coherent

PROBLEMS	INTERVENTIONS	TIME	PLAN	OUTCOME
① Potential altered nutrition: less than body requirements	maintain high-calorie, low-residue, high-protein diet; Reduce high calcium and gas-producing foods; Provide balanced meals; morning and evening supplements		Morning Care	Tol. well
		0700	Breakfast	ate entire meal
		0815	Commode	soft formed stool
		0900	Bath, Cath Care,	
		0945	ROM	
			up in wheelchair	Tolerated well
② Potential for disuse syndrome related to effects of immobility	exercise to tolerance; avoid fatigue. ROM; Turn and reposition q 1 hr.; up in wheelchair B.I.D.; encourage self-care activities to tolerance	1030	6 ℥ High Cal drink	
		1045	Returned to Bed	
		1130	Positioned on Rt side	
			Positioned on Back	
③ alteration in bowel elimination: constipation	Stool Softener, Glycerine Suppositories, enemas, PRN. Check for BM q 3 days	1230	Lunch	½ tuna sand/Tea
			up in wheelchair	
		1330	Returned to Bed	
④ Potential for infection related to indwelling Foley catheter	Routine catheter care; Change per routine schedule	1430	Positioned on left side.	
			Watching T.V.	
		1500		
⑤ Self-concept disturbance related to effects of limitations	encourage verbalization of feelings and fears. encourage independence. Be positive and reassuring			

DAILY SUMMARY
Diet and supplements taken fairly well. activity tolerated. Muscles soft but some tone. Soft formed stool. Expressed frustration during transfers from bed to wheelchair. Enjoys reading and watching T.V. Seems to be gaining some confidence in transfer activities

Visit Date ______
Nursing Supervisor Report
Pt. Last Name, First Initial Mitchell, D.
Employee Signature Ruthy Chek, CNA

Joint Visit in Home ______
Conference ______
Patient's personal care and comfort measures by home aide are: superior ___; good ___; satisfactory ___; need improvement ___;
Services provided were appropriate ___; inappropriate ___.

Comments

Figure 5–3 Sample client care plan.

and short-term goals for the home health agency's period of care for the individual. Client-focused goals must be established to provide the health care team with a communication tool specific to each client. This includes the HCA who is expected to have an understanding of the goals and the ability to observe the client's progress in reaching these goals.

The HCA is the health care provider most often in the home and who communicates with the client and the family. Many times, important information is obtained during these one-on-one personal care visits. The HCA who specializes in the care of the client requiring rehabilitation should have an increased knowledge and awareness of the problems that could slow down the process of reaching the client's goals. It is important for the specially trained HCA to:

1. Know each client's individual goals and expected outcomes.
2. Understand the possible problems that might hinder the recovery process.
3. Report these problems/changes to the supervisor so the nurse, PT, OT, or physician can decide a course of action.
4. Know that there are usually several short-term goals necessary to achieve the long-term one.

The HCA should not be concerned with setting goals since that is a nursing function. The HCA should, however, be aware of the goals because as a specialist caring for the client requiring rehabilitation, he or she will be an important part of the team working to achieve the expected goals in the period of time allowed by Medicare or the insurance company paying for this client's home health care program.

expected outcomes   the hoped-for results of short- and long-term goals

The most important aspect of setting short- and long-term goals is to determine the **expected outcomes** of these goals for the client. Nursing care plans are structured so that the nurse and physician begin the plan of care by first establishing the outcomes which are defined as:

> Statements of client/family/caregiver behaviors that can be measured and observed during the process of care. They should have a target date of accomplishment based on the individual client and that client's expected progress.

payors of home care   Medicare, HMOs, or any insurance company that covers the client's health care expenses

The **payors of home care** for the client (the insurance company or Medicare) require that the client's records include goals and expected outcomes, and that these be evaluated every week or two to confirm that they are being met. Lack of progress toward expected outcomes must be documented and explained by the nurse and HCA so that payments for visits are not stopped or questioned.

Helpful Hints: Medicare requires HCAs to be supervised by an RN in the client's home every two weeks (the supervisory visit). This is to ensure that appropriate care is being given.

The nursing care plan and the HCA care plan must reflect the course of progress or lack of progress. The nursing care plan is created, evaluated, and updated by the nurse. The HCA care plan involves both the nurse and the home care aide working together as a team.

DOCUMENTATION

documentation the written account of care given to a client

The written account of all activities, procedures carried out, and observations made when health caregivers are in the client's home is known as **documentation**. The client's record, or chart, contains documentation from all members of the care team including the nurse, physician, therapists, and the HCA. The daily visit form has space for documentation for each and every treatment, procedure, and observation. The client's record is a legal document, and the following shows a few examples of why careful and accurate recording is essential.

1. The client's record is written evidence of the care given, the client's response, and the outcome of the care.
2. The client's record reflects changes in orders and in the client's condition so that all members of the health care team can keep current.
3. The client's record is a communication tool upon which the plan for care is evaluated and updated.
4. The client's record is a written document required by insurance companies and regulatory agencies to validate the care given.
5. The client's record may be used in a court to prove that care was given and observations documented.
6. The client's record in home care is the basis for reimbursement or payment for care provided.

Every agency has its own types of records and forms. The specially trained HCA should receive proper orientation concerning the paperwork in the agency and become familiar with the documentation policies of his or her employer. Some of the forms the HCA might use are:

- ADL sheets
- daily visit forms
- graph sheets for TPRs
- HCA care plan
- client information sheet

Helpful Hints: The nurse has been called the "heart of home care" and the HCA the "heartbeat" by the National Association of Home Care.

The HCA spends more time with the client than any other member of the health care team and should be the one to observe the client for changes in condition, especially if the changes are negative. The HCA is the eyes and ears of the nurse and it is his or her responsibility to observe, document, and report everything the nurse needs to know to manage the case (see Figure 5–4).

Resident's Actions	What the HCA Will Report
agitating other residents	3:00 AM out of bed, talking to roommates, attempting to get them out of bed
confused	2:10 AM states over and over that he "wants to go to Maywood to see his mother."
disoriented	1:00 AM states "I want to go to church today because it is Sunday."
combative	9:30 PM hit nursing assistant 2x on upper arm with fist when nursing assistant attempted to change incontinent pad.
uncooperative	1:00 PM refused to get up from chair when nursing assistant tried to take to bathroom.
verbally abusive	2:20 PM called resident in next bed a "stupid, ignorant idiot."
physically abusive	10:00 AM scratched nursing assistant on face when bed was being changed.

Figure 5–4 Example of a documented observation of a client's behavior.

signs client changes that can be seen, felt, heard, or smelled

symptoms client's stated complaints

The HCA reports **signs** (changes seen, heard, felt, or smelled) and **symptoms** (complaints the client describes) to the supervisor. In addition, when the HCA reports to the supervisor, he or she must also document the same information in written form on the client's record. Figure 5–5 shows an example of a daily visit form developed to guide the HCA through the procedures that are to be done on each visit.

Some questions the HCA might ask the client in order to obtain more information before reporting to the supervisor include the following:

- What is the problem (pain, weakness, and the like)?
- Where is the problem (the client should point to where the problem is exactly)?
- Has the client had this problem before, and if so, when?
- Did the client receive any treatment that makes it worse or better (heat, ice, or Tylenol®, for example)?

The HCA should look for the following when observing their rehabilitation clients:

- Are there changes in skin status (breakdown, reddened areas, bruises, sores, bleeding, cuts)?
- Are there changes in walking (limping, weakness, unsteadiness, paralysis, shuffle, balance problems)?
- Is there pain with movement?
- Does the client have swelling in the limbs or joints?
- Is there a deformity or permanent misshaping of a body part?
- Is an extremity hot or cold?
- Does the client have a functional loss?

Name _____	No: _____	Diagnosis: _____
Home Care Aide: _____		Date of visit: _____
Date of Discharge: _____	Nurse: _____	

Routine Care:	Date:	Documentation:	Sign:
I. Observe Extremities			
A. Temperature			
B. Color			
C. Numbness			
D. Pain			
E. Ulcerations			
F. Tingling			
II. Observe Skin			
A. Reddened areas			
B. Positioning for pressure points			
C. Ulcerations/blisters			
D. Wound			
III. Observe/assist Nutrition			
A. Adequate fluid intake and output			
B. Fiber diet for bowel training			
C. Encourage/restriction fluids for bladder training			
D. Special diet			
IV. Observe/assist Home Maintainance			
A. Patient totally dependent			
B. Patient needs some assistance			
C. Patient independent (10–100%) _____			
D. Self-care			
V. Observe/assist Exercise/Activity Level			
A. PT exercise as ordered			
B. OT or ST exercise as ordered			
C. ROM exercises			
1. Passive			
2. Active			
3. Assistive			
D. Patient diability level (10–100%) _____			
VI. Observe/assist Ambulation			
A. Safety precautions			
B. Visual problems			
C. Unsteady gait			
D. Assisting devices			
E. Environment			
VII. Observe/assist Personal Care			
A. Bathing			
B. Oral care			
C. Hair care			
D. Shaving			
E. Nail care			
VIII. Observe/assist Elimination			
A. Incontinent			
B. Constipation			
C. Diarrhea			
D. Frequency/burning on urination			
E. Adequate/inadequate fluid intake			
IX. Observe Mental Status			
A. Depression			
B. Confusion			
C. Forgetfulness			
D. State of agitation			
E. Stress			
F. Oriented			
G. Impulsiveness			
H. Activity			

Specific Treatments/Procedures:	Date:	Documentation:	Sign:
Skin Care			
Positionioning/Repositioning			
Bowel and Bladder Training			
Gait Training			
Assistive Devices Training			
Return to Self-care Training			
Reinforcement of prescribed Exercise Regimen			
ROM Exercises			
Reinforcement of Speech Exercises			
Logging of Intake and Output			

Figure 5–5 HCA Visit Form for Rehabilitation (Courtesy of Health Education, Inc.)

- Does the client experience shaking, twitching, or numbness in the arms or legs?
- Are there changes in eye status (sensitivity to light, double vision, fixed pupils)?
- Does the client complain of headache or is there an observable change in mental status (slow to respond, confused, anxious, excessively fatigued)?
- Are there any changes in bodily waste elimination (bladder or bowel incontinence or painful urination or defecation)?

There are some general rules basic to all documentation. They include the following:

1. Recording should be descriptive with a note written about each complaint or problem.
2. Descriptive words instead of general terms such as "normal" or "good" should be used.
3. Writing should be neat.
4. Recording should be done in black ink.
5. Recording should begin with the date and time and end with a signature and title.
6. Recording should show the time a change was noticed and in long-term cases, a progress note at least every two hours.
7. Use quotation marks when quoting the client's symptoms.
8. All attempts to report to the supervisor should be carefully documented. If a message is left, write a note on the record describing with whom you spoke, the date, and the time.
9. Errors should not be erased. Draw a line through the wrong entry, "error" written, and place your initials next to it.
10. Use only those abbreviations accepted by the HCA's agency.
11. The HCA should only chart his or her own observations and activities, not those of another HCA. The HCA's signature legally states that he or she did the procedure and documented it.
12. If a new page is added, the client's name must be on each page as well as the time, date, and a signature.

The following is an example of how documentation for a situation involving a rehabilitation client should be handled by the HCA.

Helpful Hints: The HCA's notes should reflect that person's level of professionalism as well as an attitude of caring and concern. Write carefully and accurately.

The HCA arrives at Mrs. Edna Cromwell's home at 8 AM to find that she is still in bed, even though yesterday she had gotten up unassisted to the bedside commode. The client is six weeks postoperative from a hip pinning and has been progressing well both in activity and in strength. She tells you, "I got up during the night to go to the bathroom on the commode chair, and lost my balance. I slipped, but didn't fall on the floor. I did hurt myself though because I have a lot of pain where my operation was done."

The HCA should:

- take vital signs
- observe the client's body, especially around the incision area
- report the complaints to the supervisor immediately

The HCA's report should be documented as follows:

8:00 AM—Upon arrival, found Mrs. Edna Cromwell lying in bed with an expression of pain and crying. Client states, "I got up during the night to go to the bathroom on the commode chair, and lost my balance. I slipped, but didn't fall on the floor. I did hurt myself because I have a lot of pain where my operation was done." VS—140/90, TPR 98.2-90-24. Supervisor notified of client's condition.

8:15 AM—Bath given to client in bed. Supervisor awaiting response from physician and skilled nurse due at this home when orders received.

9:00 AM—Nurse arrived with new orders. Care plan updated. Cold compresses applied to left hip. No bruises, swelling, or redness noted at this time.

10:00 AM—Client states, "Pain is gone and I feel much better."

Helpful Hints: The agency is paid by the insurance company for the visit. The client and the HCA's signatures are legal proof that the visit was indeed completed.

HOME CARE AIDE CARE PLAN AND DAILY VISIT FORM

The contents of the HCA care plan for the rehabilitation client is determined by the nurse on the case based on the condition of the patient and the physician's orders. The nurse can make the HCA care plan individualized for each client based on specific nursing diagnoses, the client's activities of daily living, that client's goals, and the expected outcomes. As the rehabilitation client's condition improves or changes, the nurse continually updates the care plan in the "changes" section. The HCA care plan is divided into nine main areas to which special attention is paid on each visit. These include:

- extremities
- skin
- nutrition
- home maintenance
- exercise/activity level
- ambulation

- personal care
- elimination
- mental status

In addition to these routine areas of concern, the nurse would most likely emphasize:

- skin care
- prevention of deformities
- reinforcement of the client's exercise program
- gait training
- safety precautions
- bowel and bladder training
- observation of changes in rehabilitation status
- reinforcement of speech program
- safe ambulation and transfers
- measures to reestablish self-care

In order to accommodate the increased HCA activities and documentation, it has become necessary for the care plan to be specific to each rehabilitation client. There are observation requirements for each visit and specific procedures for rehabilitative care that are performed on some clients and not on others. The care plan, therefore, is divided into those routine tasks that should be done on every visit and those which the nurse instructs the HCA to do for that specific client on that specific visit. The HCA care plan and daily visit form are important communication tools and it is important that the HCA make it a part of the routine documentation.

Helpful Hints: Never hesitate to ask the nurse or supervisor a question about the client. They want you to be informed.

REVIEW QUESTIONS

1. The _____ _____ is the basis for the nursing care plan and HCA care plan.
2. The _____ is the health care person who communicates most frequently with the client.
3. Two important aspects involved when the HCA and nurse act as a team are _____ and _____ .
4. Which of the following is *not* included in the HCA care plan?
   a. nutrition
   b. activity
   c. PT goals
   d. personal care

5. Choose the area or areas of concern that should be emphasized in caring for rehabilitation clients:
   a. self-care
   b. skin care
   c. safety
   d. all of the above
6. True or False? All clients who require rehabilitation need bowel and bladder training.
7. True or False? Clients should be encouraged to do as much for themselves as possible and allowed to do so even if it takes more time.
8. True or False? Some clients might not remember their progress from one day to the next.
9. True or False? The client's goals and expected outcomes must be considered on a twenty-four-hour basis to obtain the best results.
10. True or False? The physician writes the treatment plan.
11. True or False? The HCA writes the HCA Care Plan.
12. Unscramble the following key term from the chapter: xpeetdce motusoce _____ _____

CHAPTER 6

Client Care

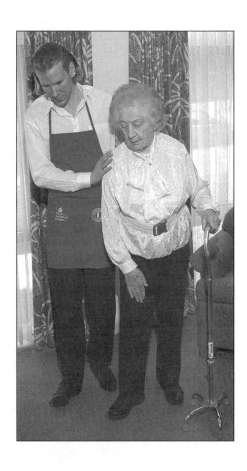

OBJECTIVES

Upon reading this chapter and completing the review questions, the home care aide should be able to:

1. Understand range of motion exercises and their guidelines and benefits.

2. Define the importance of positioning the client and the use of supportive devices.

3. Describe five types of gait training and the methods used for special clients.

4. Describe decubitus ulcer prevention and all aspects of skin care.

5. Describe bowel and bladder training techniques and indications.

6. Define personal care as it applies to rehabilitation and disabled clients.
7. Define home maintenance and the HCA's role and function.

KEY TERMS

amputation	decubitus ulcers
bladder training	functional limitations
body mechanics	gait training
bowel training	home maintenance

INTRODUCTION

The excellent care of the client requiring rehabilitation by the HCA includes several important aspects which must be discussed in more depth. These are exercises, positioning, gait training, skin care, special aspects of personal care, and bowel and bladder training.

RANGE OF MOTION EXERCISES

Range of motion exercises are done to prevent joint contractures and maintain or increase joint mobility. The HCA who has been trained to do ROM exercises should perform this procedure in one of four ways:

1. Passive ROM in which the client does not participate and movements are done solely by the HCA.
2. Active-assistive ROM in which the client participates but still requires the HCA's assistance.
3. Active ROM in which the client performs all of the movements and the HCA observes and records the procedure.
4. Resistive ROM in which the client performs the movements with weights.

Refer to Client Care Procedure 1, below, to perform passive range of motion exercises.

CLIENT CARE PROCEDURE

1 Performing Passive Range of Motion Exercises

PURPOSE

- To increase muscle tone and strength in the client's body
- To restore function to injured parts of the body
- To prevent joint stiffness and contractures

CLIENT CARE PROCEDURE, *continued*

1   **Performing Passive Range of Motion Exercises**

NOTE: Do not perform the exercises until you have received instructions specific for your client's joints. When possible, support the extremity above and below the joints being exercised. If the client shows pain or discomfort, stop the exercise and document it. The head can be exercised if specifically ordered by the physical therapist. Exercises can be done in bed or in the chair. It is important to keep the client covered or clothed to prevent unnecessary exposure during the procedure.

PROCEDURE

1. Wash your hands.
2. Read any special instructions for the exercises for your client.
3. Tell client what you plan to do. Ask client to assist as much as possible.
4. Exercise the shoulder—Supporting the upper and lower arms, exercise the shoulder joint. Abduct (away from the body) the entire arm out at right angles to the body (see Figure 6–1A). Then adduct the arm (bring back to the midline of the body) to the center of the client's body (see Figure 6–1B).
5. Exercise the elbow—Bend elbow, keeping the arm close to the body. Bring the fingers to touch the shoulder (see Figure 6–2A). Lower the fingers to touch the bed (see Figure 6–2B)

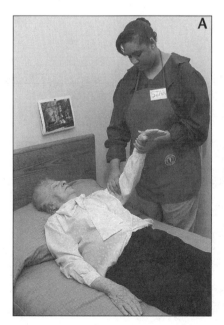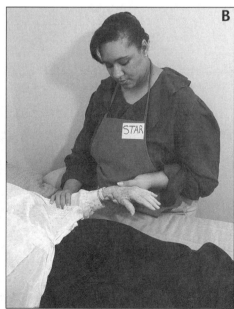

Figure 6–1   Exercising the shoulder joint

1   Performing Passive Range of Motion Exercises

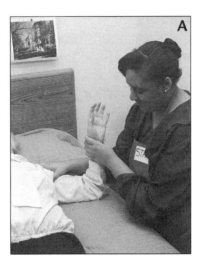
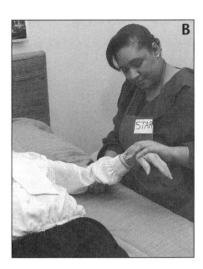

Figure 6–2 Excercising the elbow

6. Exercise the forearm—Bring the arm out to the side. Rest it on the bed. Take the client's hand and rotate the arm, palm up and palm down (See Figures 6–3A and B).

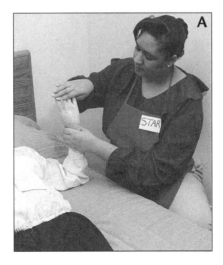
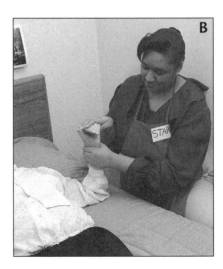

Figure 6–3 Exercising the forearm

1   Performing Passive Range of Motion Exercises

7. Exercise the wrist and fingers—Take the client's hand and move the hand forward and back (see Figure 6–4A and B). Move the hand from side to side. Curl the client's fingers and straighten them (Figures 6–4C and D). Spread the fingers apart and rotate the thumb. Touch all fingers to thumb (see Figure 6–4E).

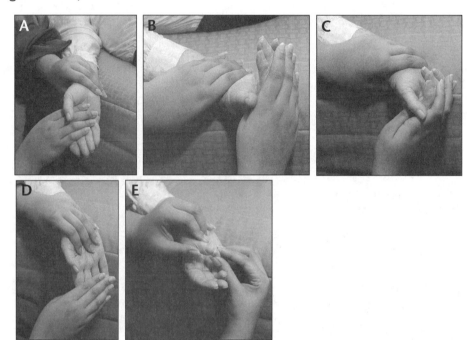

Figure 6–4 Exercising the wrist and fingers

8. Exercise the knee and hip—Keep the client lying on his or her back. Bend the knee and raise it to the chest (see Figure 6–5). Bring the leg out to the side and back. Cross one leg over the other. Allow the leg to rest on the bed with the knee straight and the heel resting on the bed. Rotate the leg inward and outward.

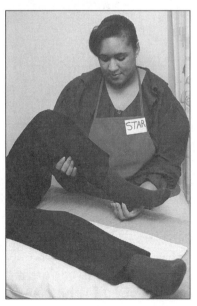

Figure 6–5 Exercising the knee and hip

1 Performing Passive Range of Motion Exercises

9. Exercise the ankle—Bend client's knee slightly and support lower leg with one hand. With the other hand, bend client's foot downward (plantar flexion) and then bend client's foot toward the body (dorsiflexion) (see Figures 6–6A and B). With client's legs extended on the bed, place both hands on the client's foot and move foot inward and then outward.

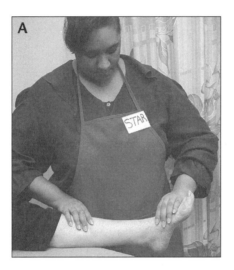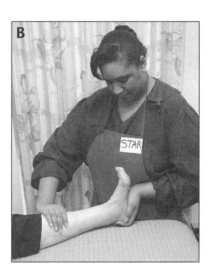

Figure 6–6 Exercising the ankle and foot

10. Exercise the toes—Bend (flexion) and straighten (extension) each toe. Perform abduction and adduction with each toe as you did with the fingers.
11. Go to the client's other side and repeat movements for each joint.
12. Wash hands.
13. Document the completion of the exercises and the client's reactions.

ROM exercises are usually performed with the client in bed, but can be done with the client standing. The benefits of performing ROM exercises include keeping the muscles strong and the joints working, preventing deformities and spasticity, promoting blood circulation, improving mobility and coordination, and enhancing the client's self-esteem. In some cases, the PT Assistant or the OT performs the ROM exercises for the client.

ROM exercises are performed as prescribed in the treatment plan and described in the care plan and are usually done during

functional limitations the client's level of ambulation and activity

or after the bath and again later in the day. Some clients may require ROM exercises as often as every four hours. The guidelines to follow for ROM exercises are:

- The HCA should always check the care plan and/or supervisor's instructions for the client's **functional limitations**.
- Each exercise should be done five times unless otherwise instructed.
- The joints to be exercised should be specifically ordered.
- When appropriate, the HCA should begin at the head and work toward the feet in an organized manner.
- The HCA should be careful not to expose the client during the exercises (put underpants or pajama bottoms on the client).
- The HCA should encourage the client to do as much as he or she can, if that is ordered by the physician or nurse.
- The HCA should never force an extremity past a comfortable point.
- It the client complains of pain, the HCA should stop the exercise and report to the supervisor.
- The arm or leg being exercised should be supported.
- The HCA should use slow, smooth, gentle movements.
- If the joint or extremity appears to be swollen, red, or painful, the HCA should stop the exercise and report to the supervisor.
- If the client refuses to do the exercises, the HCA should report immediately to the supervisor.
- The HCA should document what exercises were done, the time, any observations, and how the client responded.

REPOSITIONING THE CLIENT

Repositioning the client is an important procedure to ensure comfort and to prevent contractures. Good body alignment for the client is important. The back should be straight and in alignment during transfers or while the client is in any position. The HCA should know if there are any problems the client has or positions that are not appropriate. When turning the client, a drawsheet should be used to prevent friction on the skin. Shearing or forcing the skin to move in an opposite direction causes skin breakdown and should be avoided. Client Care Procedures 2, 3, 4, and 5 show how to position the client in four positions.

2 Positioning the Client in Supine Position

PURPOSE

- To make the client more comfortable
- Assist the body to function more efficiently

PROCEDURE

1. Wash your hands.
2. Tell client what you plan to do.
3. Place pillow under the client's head about two inches above the level of the bed. The pillow should extend slightly under the shoulders (see Figure 6–7).

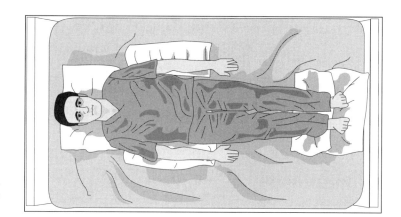

Figure 6–7 A client in supine position. The head may be elevated slightly with a pillow and the arms supported with pillows for comfort. A pillow is placed under the feet to prevent pressure on the heels.

4. Have client's arms extend straight out with palms of the hands flat on the bed. The arms can be supported by pillows or covered foam pads placed under the forearms and extending from just above the elbows to the ends of the fingers.
5. Place a small pillow or rolled towel along the side of the client's thighs and tuck part of the support under the thigh, ensuring that the part under the thighs is smooth. This maintains alignment of the hips and thighs and helps prevent the hips from rotating outward or externally.
6. Place a pillow under the back of the ankle to relieve pressure on the heels.
7. Wash your hands.
8. Document the time, position change, and the client's reaction.

CLIENT CARE PROCEDURE

3   Positioning the Client in Lateral Side-laying Position

PURPOSE

- To provide client comfort
- To relieve pressure on body parts

PROCEDURE

1. Wash your hands.
2. Tell client what you plan to do.
3. Go to the side of the bed opposite the direction from which you are planning to turn the client.
4. Cross the client's arms over the chest. Place your arm under the client's neck and shoulders. Place your other arm under the client's midback. Move the upper part of the client's body toward you.
5. Place one arm under the client's waist and the other under the thighs. Move the lower part of the client's body toward you.
6. Turn client to opposite side. Pull shoulder that is touching the bed slightly toward you. Pull buttock that is touching the bed slightly toward you. Place pillow under back and buttocks. Place bottom leg in extension and flex upper leg. Place small folded blanket or pillow between the upper and lower legs.
7. Place pillow under the client's head. Rotate the upper arm to bring it up to the pillow with the palm facing up. Place the other arm on a pillow that extends from above the elbow to the fingers. Extend the fingers.
8. Check the client's position to see if the body is in good vertical alignment (see Figure 6–8).

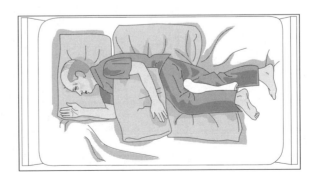

Figure 6–8 Lateral/side-laying position

9. Wash your hands.
10. Document time, change of position, and client's reaction.

4   Positioning the Client in Prone Position

PURPOSE

- To relieve pressure on body parts
- To provide client comfort

NOTE: Most elderly clients are not able to lie on their stomach and do not like to be in this position for long periods of time. Before turning a dependent client to the prone position, make sure client's arms are straight down at sides to avoid injury while turning. Never leave an older client in this position more than 15 to 20 minutes.

PROCEDURE

1. Wash your hands.
2. Tell client what you plan to do.
3. Turn client on abdomen. Check to see if spine is straight and face is turned to one side or the other.
4. Legs should be extended and arms flexed and brought up to either side of head.
5. A small pillow can be placed under the abdomen, especially for women because this reduces pressure against their breasts. An alternate method is to roll a small towel and place it under the shoulders to reduce pressure.
6. Place another pillow under lower legs to prevent pressure on toes (see Figure 6–9). Client can also be moved to foot of bed so that the feet extend over the mattress.

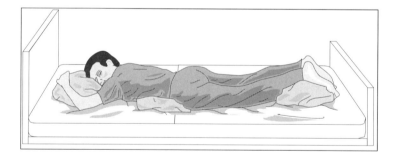

Figure 6–9   Prone position

7. Wash your hands.
8. Document time, position change, and client's reaction.

5 Positioning the Client in Fowler's Position

PURPOSE

- To provide client comfort
- To aid in breathing
- To position client so that he or she can engage in activities such as eating, reading, watching television, or visiting with a family member or friend.

NOTE: If the client is weak or frail, the sitting position may be hard for the client to maintain. Supporting the client with pillows helps the client maintain the sitting position.

PROCEDURE

1. Wash your hands.
2. Tell the client what you plan to do.
3. Check to see if the client's spine and legs are straight and that he or she is in the middle of the bed.
4. Support client's head and neck with one, two, or three pillows. If client has a hospital bed, raise bed to a 45-degree angle.
5. Knees may be flexed and supported with small pillows (see Figure 6–10).

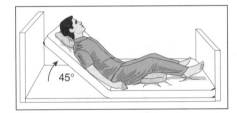

Figure 6–10 Fowler's position

6. Pillows may be placed under each arm from elbows to fingertips to support shoulders.
7. Place pillow or padded footboard against feet.
8. Wash your hands.
9. Document time, position change, and client's reaction.

Helpful Hints: Some agencies require the HCA to wear a back belt when repositioning the client when there is a risk of injury to the aide.

The client's posture as well as that of the HCA are both important. Many clients can help with the moving process. However, the HCA may have to reposition clients who cannot help. In this case, it might require two persons to perform the positioning procedure. The family caregiver can assist the HCA when necessary. The HCA should have a plan for positioning the client and have pillows and other devices ready before beginning the procedure.

body mechanics   correct and
safe use of the body for work

Before moving the client, the HCA should review the principles of **body mechanics** which include:

* Correct posture to make lifting, pulling, and pushing easier
  (see Figure 6–11A and B).
* Keep the back straight, and use the thigh muscles, not the
  back muscles (see Figure 6-12).
* Turn with a pivoting motion, never from the waist (see Figure
  6–13A and B).
* Hold heavy objects close to the body (see Figure 6–14). Push,
  pull, or roll rather than lift.
* Keep feet approximately 12 inches apart for proper body support (see Figure 6–15).
* Use verbal signals to let the client and other workers know
  when the move begins.

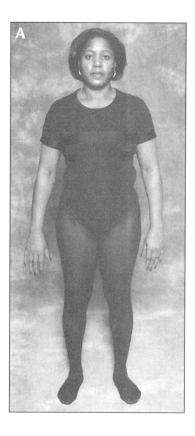

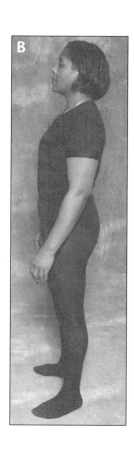

Figure 6–11   Correct standing position—A. Front view, B. Side view

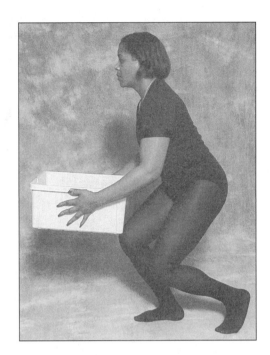

Figure 6–12 The correct way to maintain balance when picking up an object is to bend from the hips and knees.

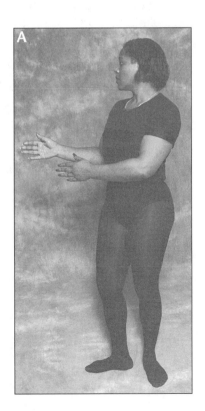
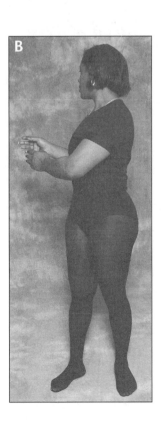

Figure 6–13 A. Pivot instead of twisting—B. Avoid twisting the body

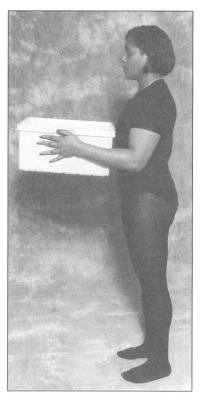

Figure 6–14 Hold objects close to the body

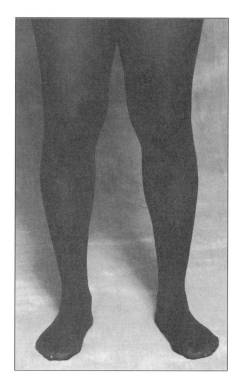

Figure 6–15 Keep feet apart

Helpful Hints: Practice good body mechanics to prevent back injury and to assist clients properly.

Repositioning of clients is done when they are lying in bed or sitting in chairs. Proper repositioning prevents complications such as pressure sores and body deformities. The following are general guidelines for lifting and moving clients:

• The HCA should know if there are any special considerations involving the client before beginning a move and he or she should discuss repositioning with the supervisor.

• Have a written plan so that positions can be varied during a twenty-four-hour period.

• Always tell the client what is going to happen so that he or she can help as much as possible if the treatment plan permits.

• Be careful not to touch painful areas.

• Be gentle and use slow, smooth movements. Stop if the client evidences pain.

• Allow the client periods of rest during the procedure, if necessary.

Supportive devices might be needed to keep the body in proper alignment. Some of these devices include footboards to prevent foot drop, special foot devices to help maintain foot position (see Figure 6–16), bedboards to make the mattress firm, trochanter rolls to prevent the hips and legs from turning out-

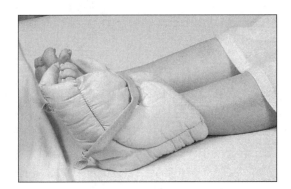

Figure 6–16 Special foot devices keep the foot in the correct position

ward (see Figure 6–17), hand rolls to prevent contractures of the hands and wrists, and bed cradles to keep linens off the feet (see Figure 6–18).

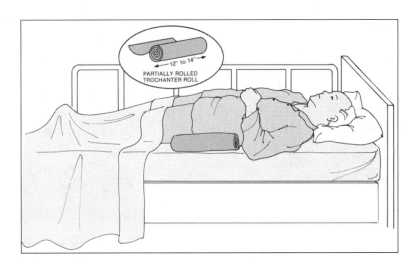

Figure 6–17 Trochanter roll in place

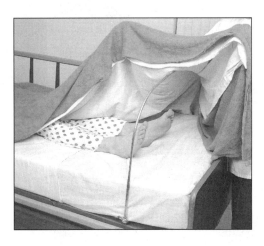

Figure 6–18 A bed cradle keeps sheets from putting pressure on the feet.

When positioning a client, the HCA should have several pillows (usually three or four) in various sizes to support the head or the back and to keep the client from rolling off to the side. Rolled towels or blankets can be used in the home between the legs or ankles and between bones to prevent friction. They also can be used as trochanter rolls. Footboards can be purchased or blankets and boxes placed at the foot of the bed. All clients who are on a repositioning program should have turning sheets and/or draw sheets. Turning schedules usually require position changes at least every two hours.

GAIT TRAINING

gait training   teaching the client the proper gait (walk) with assistive devices

Gait training must be ordered by the physician and planned by the physical therapist. However, the HCA is often involved in reinforcement and practice of gait training. Assistive devices involved in gait training are crutches, canes, and walkers which come in many shapes and sizes and which we have already discussed under the heading "rehabilitation equipment." Gait training is a rehabilitative exercise to assist the client improve ambulation in the process of returning him or her to the highest possible level of activity.

Helpful Hints: Finding help in the home might be a problem. HCAs, however, should not hesitate to ask the family to assist in situations in order to avoid client falls or injuries. When in doubt, HCAs should not put themselves or their client at risk.

Safety is an important feature and the HCA should have help, particularly if the client is very weak. The area in which the client walks must be cleared of clutter and scatter rugs and there should be no wet areas on the floor. Assistive devices should have safety features such as proper fittings, nonskid tips, and be adapted to the client's extremity weaknesses. A gait belt should be used for those clients who have a high risk of falling. Figure 6–19A shows how to put on a gait belt properly and Figure 6–19B shows how to use it properly.

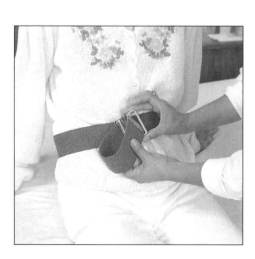

Figure 6–19A   A belt is put on the client's waist by first slipping the end through the opening with the "teeth." Insert two fingers between the belt and the client's waist to ensure that the belt is not too tight.

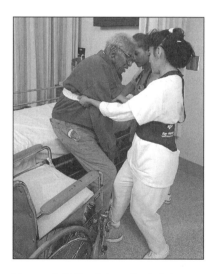

Figure 6–19B   A transfer belt is used to hold onto the client during transfer.

Figures 6–20 and 6–21 show how the HCA should support the client when gait training.

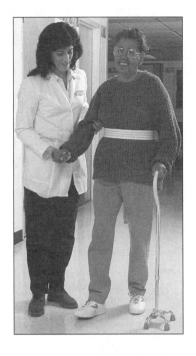

Figure 6–20 Many clients need assistance with walking to prevent them from falling.

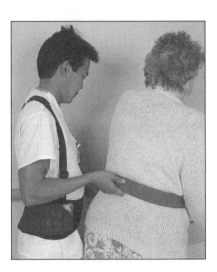

Figure 6–21 This transfer belt is used to hold onto the client while she is ambulating.

There are five basic gaits and the method used depends on the client's individual problems and condition. The five gaits are:

1. The four-point alternating gait, used when the client can bear weight on both feet.
2. The three-point gait, used when the client can bear weight on only one foot and the problem leg does not touch the ground.
3. The two-point gait, used when the client can bear weight on both feet.
4. The swing-to-crutch gait, used when the client can bear some weight on both feet but uses the upper arm muscles as strength.
5. The swing-through-crutch gait which requires strong upper arm muscles to lift and swing the body through.

A cane is used when there is weakness on one side of the body to help with balance and to support the client. There are one-, three-, and four-pointed canes. The single-tip cane is held on the strong side (if the left leg is weak, the cane is held in the right hand).

A walker is a four-point walking aid which gives the client the most support. The walker is picked up and moved in front of the client. In addition, some walkers have wheels. Refer to Client Care Procedure 6 for assisting the client to walk with a walker, crutches, or a cane.

6   Assisting the Client to Walk with Crutches, Walker, or Cane

PURPOSE

- To provide support and maintain balance as client walks.

NOTE: There are three basic walking patterns. With a nonweight-bearing pattern, all the weight is placed on the arms and uninvolved leg. Partial weight-bearing means that minimal weight is placed on the toes. However, most weight is still on the arms and the uninvolved leg.

To walk in a nonweight-bearing pattern, the client uses crutches (see Figure 6–22). The physical therapist measures the client to select the correct length of crutches. The therapist also teaches the client how to walk with them.

To walk in a partial weight-bearing pattern, the client can use crutches but often uses a walker instead. The walker is a curved metal frame with four legs. It is a walking aid that gives maximum stability as the client moves. The client steps forward while holding onto the walker with both hands. Some walkers have wheels so that the client does not have to lift up the walker between steps (see Figure 6–23).

A cane is used when the client is strong enough to bear full weight on both legs. A standard cane should not be used as a weight-bearing aid. A special cane with four short legs, called a quad cane, is designed to bear a small amount of weight only (see Figure 6–24). A cane is primarily used for balance. Check rubber tips on canes, walkers, and crutches as they wear out quickly if used on sidewalks.

Always have client wear good supportive shoes with nonskid soles. Instruct clients to pick up feet and not to look at feet but straight ahead.

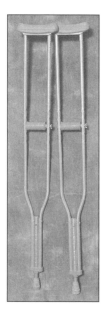

Figure 6–22   Crutches

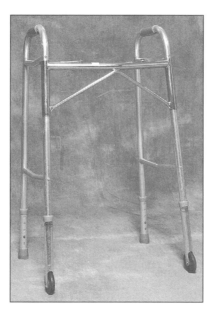

Figure 6–23   Walker with small wheels

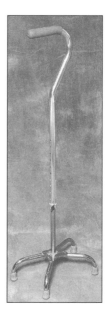

Figure 6–24   Four-point (quad) cane

6   Assisting the Client to Walk with Crutches, Walker, or Cane

PROCEDURE

1. Wash your hands. Apply transfer belt unless instructed not to.
2. Always walk on the client's weak side.
3. Walk slightly behind the client holding onto the transfer belt from behind.
4. For the client using crutches, hold on to the transfer belt if the client feels uncomfortable using the crutches (see Figure 6–25 A and B).

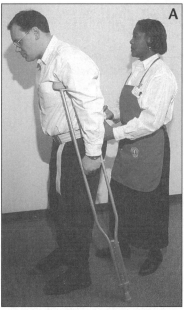
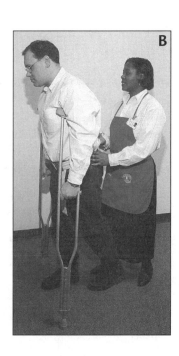

Figure 6–25   Walking with crutches

5. For the client using a walker, instruct the client to place the walker firmly before walking. If the client is strong enough, the walker and the weaker leg can be moved forward at the same time.
6. For the client using a cane (see Figure 6–26A and B), instruct him or her to hold the cane in the hand opposite the weaker leg. For example, if the right ankle has been injured, the client should hold the cane in the left hand.

CLIENT CARE PROCEDURE. *continued*

6   Assisting the Client to Walk with Crutches, Walker, or Cane

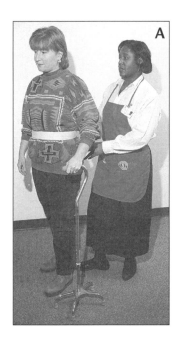
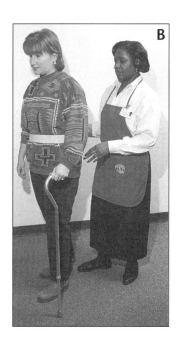

Figure 6–26   Use of various types of canes

7. Balance is a judgmental situation. If the client has poor balance, the aide should support the weak side. If the client has good balance and can walk without assistive devices, the aide should use a transfer belt for safety reasons.

8. Wash your hands at completion of the procedure.

9. Document how far the client walked and client's reaction.

SKIN CARE

Skin care is given to rehabilitation clients to prevent breakdown of the skin which could lead to decubitus ulcers. When there is pressure, shearing, or friction on the skin, breakdown occurs. Because clients requiring rehabilitation have impaired mobility, their risk is higher for **decubitus ulcers**. Other contributing factors include lack of cleanliness, moisture (such as perspiration or urine), incontinence, and soap left on the skin. The skin breaks down in four stages:

Stage I—Redness lasting longer than 30 minutes after pressure is removed. The area may be warm to the touch.

Stage II—The skin is reddened and has a blister or broken area on the surface.

decubitus ulcers   skin breakdown over body areas due to pressure or friction

Stage III—Layers of the skin have been destroyed and may or may not be infected.

Stage IV—The skin is gone and the ulcer is deep into the muscle and bone.

Figure 6–27A, B, C, and D shows the four stages of skin breakdown and Figure 6–28 shows the most common sites of skin breakdown.

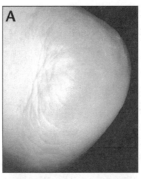
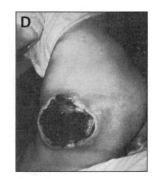
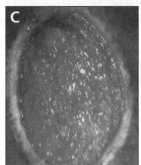

Figure 6–27 A. First indication of tissue ischemia (Stage I) is redness and heat over a pressure point such as this heel.
B. Stage II is marked by destruction of the epidermis and partial destruction of the dermis. Photo shows coccygeal (sacrum) area.
C. In Stage III, all layers of skin have been destroyed and a deep crater has been formed. Photo shows right hip.
D. In Stage IV, skin is gone and ulcer is deep into muscle and bone. (Courtesy of Emory University Hospital, Atlanta, GA).

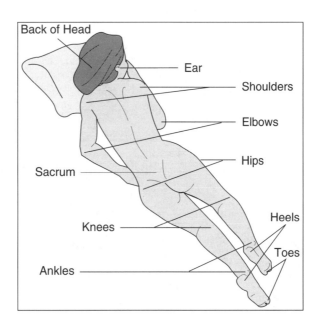

Figure 6–28 Most common sites of skin breakdown

Seven ways to prevent skin breakdown are to:

1. Remove pressure from bony areas.
2. Massage the skin surrounding the area.
3. Keep skin clean and dry.
4. Reposition the client.
5. Remove urine and feces from the skin promptly.
6. Pat skin dry instead of rubbing.
7. Give back massages.

The client's skin should be observed regularly and accurately, especially at pressure points (see Figure 6–29). The HCA should report any changes in the skin such as redness, heat, tenderness, or blisters immediately. The HCA should also keep a record of position changes. Figure 6–30 is an example of a chart used to record position changes. Incontinent clients should be checked for dryness frequently—at least every one to two hours—and measures taken to keep urine and feces off the skin by wearing protective pads or briefs. Depends® and other disposable briefs should be changed frequently. Preventative devices can be used to prevent skin breakdown such as specialty beds, specialty mattresses, sheepskin heel and elbow protectors, and bed cradles.

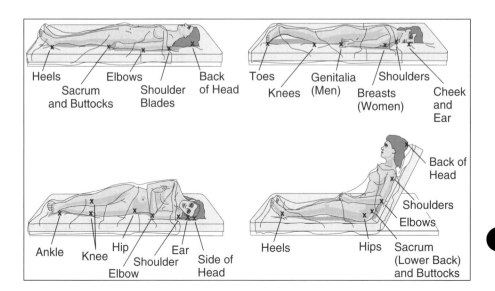

Figure 6–29 Possible pressure points

				FRAMINGHAM HOME			

POSITION-CHANGE BEDSIDE RECORD
NAME Smith. Emily   ROOM NUMBER 118 B

DATE	TIME	POSIT.	SIGNA.	DATE	TIME	POSIT.	SIGNA.
4/17	7 AM	Dorsol Recombent	JH.				
	9 AM	Left Sims	JH.				
	11 AM	Prone	JH.				

Figure 6–30 The position change record should be kept at the bedside for convenience.

Refer to Client Care Procedure 7 for special skin care and to prevent pressure sores.

CLIENT CARE PROCEDURE

7   Special Skin Care and Pressure Sores

PURPOSE

- To prevent skin breakdown resulting from pressure and skin irritations
- To use preventive devices
- To prevent friction resulting from skin being in contact with skin or bed linens

NOTE: Certain clients are at risk for the development of pressure areas leading to sores. Clients at risk are bedridden: they may be obese, very thin, diabetic, paralyzed, and/or malnourished. A home health aide's role is mainly in the prevention of pressure sore development. Once a pressure sore has developed, the nurse then comes to the client's home to treat the open area.

ASSISTIVE DEVICES TO PREVENT PRESSURE SORES

1. Air mattress—This is a mattress filled with air. It works by continuously changing the pressure areas on the client's back. One can improvise with an air mattress designed for camping instead of buying a medical air mattress.
2. Egg crate mattress—This is a mattress made from foam rubber molded into an egg crate pattern. Egg crate mattresses are inexpensive and effective in reducing pressure on the skin. One can also purchase a seat for the client to sit on during the day when up in a chair.
3. Water mattress—This is similar to a regular water mattress used in the home. The mattress is effective in reducing pressure on the skin but causes problems when transferring clients in and out of bed.
4. Gel foam cushion—This is a special cushion filled with a special solution or gel. The cushion is effective in the prevention of pressure sores for the client who sits in a wheelchair for long periods of time.

7 Special Skin Care and Pressure Sores

5. Sheepskin or lamb's wool pads for elbows and heels—Lamb's wool pads prevent pressure sores by acting as a barrier between the client's skin and the sheets.
6. Bed cradle—This is a device to keep linens off the client's legs and feet. In the home, an aide can substitute a box or other device to keep linens off the legs and feet.

SPECIAL CARE TO PREVENT PRESSURE SORES

1. Change client's position at least every two hours to reduce pressure on any one area.
2. As quickly as possible, remove feces, urine, or moisture of any kind that might be irritating to the skin.
3. Encourage clients who sit in chairs or wheelchairs to raise themselves or change position every 15 minutes to relieve pressure.
4. Encourage client to eat a high protein diet (if allowed by the physician) and to drink adequate amounts of fluids.
5. Keep bed linens clean, dry, and wrinklefree.
6. When bathing clients, use soap sparingly because soap drys skin. Keep skin well lubricated.
7. Watch for skin irritation when applying braces and splints.
8. At the first sign of a reddened area, gently massage area around the spot. Report observations to the nurse or supervisor immediately.

Helpful Hints: The HCA should always report suspicious skin areas immediately to protect the client, the agency, and themselves.

The HCA should follow the guidelines set down by the agency for special skin care programs. Cleanliness is the main objective along with careful observation and documentation. The HCA can apply special creams and ointments as directed by the nurse or the supervisor and stimulate circulation in the client's back, buttocks, and bony areas by means of gentle massage.

ASSISTING IN DRESSING THE CLIENT

Assistance in dressing the client is frequently required with rehabilitation clients. There are many dressing aids on the market which are described in Chapter 4 under "personal care devices." The client should always be encouraged to do as much as possible according to the physician's orders, the nursing care plan, and his or her limitations. Clients should be encouraged not to wear pajamas during the day, but rather to dress in their clothes to encourage a feeling of participation in a normal life.

Bedbound clients, of course, will have to be dressed or assisted to dress, by the HCA. Bedbound clients should be in hospital gowns, if possible, to make dressing and undressing easier for the workers. Bedclothes that are easily changed are best. But even clients who are bedbound can select their clothes and do as much self-care as possible.

Before assisting the clients in dressing, the HCA should have the client select his or her clothes for the day. This gives the client a feeling of control and increases self-esteem. Clothing should be clean and neat and not too loose fitting to present a safety problem for the client who has a physical limitation. Refer to Client Care Procedure 8 for dressing and undressing a client.

CLIENT CARE PROCEDURE

8   Dressing and Undressing the Client

PURPOSE

- To keep the client clean and comfortable
- To increase the client's self-image and well-being
- To reduce client's discomfort and reduce his or her risk of strain or injury

NOTE: Do not allow the client to remain in nightclothes during the day (unless the case manager states it is permitted). The client needs to know that it is daytime and to dress accordingly.

PROCEDURE

1. Wash your hands and tell the client what you plan to do.
2. Assemble clean clothing:
   undergarments
   outergarments—let clients select their own, if possible
   stockings and shoes
3. If client is able, help him or her to sit at the edge of the bed and dangle the legs. If the client is too weak to sit up, have him or her lie flat on the bed. Place a sheet or robe over the client to avoid embarrassment or chilling.
4. Assist the client in putting on undergarments. If the client has a weak leg, place weak leg in first, then the other leg. Put on outergarments in the same manner. If client can stand, pull the pants or slacks up to the waist. If the client must remain on the bed, ask the client to press his or her heels into the bed and raise the buttocks. While the client is in this position, quickly slide the pants or slacks up to the waist. Assist the client as necessary. Slacks with elastic waist are preferred as they go on easier than pants with zippers and buttons. Cotton jogging suits are becoming a very popular option for disabled or elderly clients. They are warm, easy to get off and on, and attractive. They also launder easily.
5. To dress the client in a shirt, slip, or dress, help the client place the weak arm into the sleeve first (see figure 6–31A), then the strong arm. If the dress or shirt needs to go over the head, help client place both arms into the armholes and then slip the neck of the garment over the client's head.

8   Dressing and Undressing the Client

6. To put on socks or stockings, turn each sock down to the toe end. Slide client's toe into place and, with one arm on each side of leg, pull the sock or stocking up (see Figure 6–31B). Make sure socks are smooth over the feet and legs. Put on shoes if client is to remain out of bed. Let client assist as much as possible.

Helpful Hints: It sometimes takes great patience on the part of the person assisting the client to allow him or her plenty of time without feeling rushed.

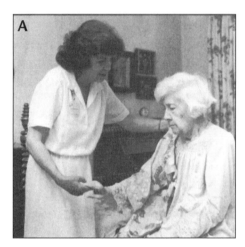

Figure 6–31A Place weak arm into sleeve first, followed by the strong arm.

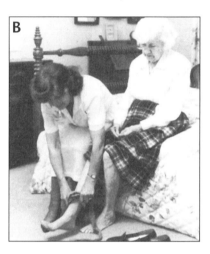

Figure 6–31B Roll stocking down to the toe, then put on foot.

7. To undress the client, simply reverse the instructions for dressing. If the client has a weak arm or leg, undress the weak limb last.
8. Wash hands.

BOWEL AND BLADDER TRAINING

Bowel and bladder training is an important rehabilitation process for clients with waste elimination dysfunction and/or incontinence. Some clients have lost all or part of their control and in some cases, the physician and the nurse may determine that bowel or bladder rehabilitation training can be useful in regaining some or all of this control. Often, incontinence can be prevented by offering the bedpan or urinal to the client on a regular basis.

For cases requiring **bowel training**, the physician may order suppositories to stimulate the rectum to produce a bowel movement. The HCA may be asked to assist the client in inserting the suppository. In addition, the HCA should observe the client's ability to control his or her bowels in terms of how long the suppository is retained before a bowel movement occurs. Occasionally, enemas are ordered as part of bowel training and the HCA should check first with the supervisor to determine the agency's

bowel training   training to restore the client's ability to control bowel movements

policy and procedure for giving enemas. States vary in their regulations which may or may not allow HCAs to give enemas. Commercially prepared enemas are usually approved for HCA use. Oil-retention enemas are commercially prepared. The client should retain the oil, in bed in a quiet position, for as long as possible. Oil enemas work best if warmed first by soaking in warm water for 30 minutes. Refer to Client Care Procedure 9 for training and retraining bowels. Refer to Client Care Procedure 10 for a method of inserting a rectal suppository. Refer to Client Care Procedure 11 for administering an enema.

CLIENT CARE PROCEDURE

9   Training and Retraining Bowels

PURPOSE

- To train a client to be continent of bowel movement
- To regulate a client to have regular bowel movements

NOTE: Constipation can result from illness, poor eating habits, drug therapy, and lack of exercise. Constipation causes the client added discomfort when it occurs in addition to other physical problems. An individualized bowel program is designed by the health care team for each client. For instance, one client can regulate the bowels by adding prune juice to the diet twice a day. Another client may need to drink daily prune juice and require a daily laxative and stool softener in addition.

Older clients can become overly "bowel conscious" and have a misconception of what normal elimination should be. The frequency of bowel movements may range from three times a day for one person to only once every two or three days for another. Therefore, the term constipation should not be used to describe a missed movement or two, but only the unusual retention of fecal matter along with infrequent or difficult passage of stony, hard stool.

Constipation is very often encountered among the elderly. If a client is unable to exercise and move about regularly, bowel action becomes sluggish. Sometimes medications, especially painkillers, can cause constipation. If a client has hemorrhoids, there may be a fear of pain and the client avoids trying to have a bowel movement. If a client does not have a bowel movement for a few days, he or she may develop an impaction, a large amount of hard stool in the lower colon or rectum. This is a very painful condition. If a client does develop an impaction, the nurse may have to remove it manually.

PROCEDURE

1. The health care team assesses prior habits of the client. If the client always had a bowel movement early in the morning, this is important to know in planning the retraining program.
2. A plan is designed and implemented. Important elements of the plan are:
   - high intake of fiber foods
   - adequate intake of liquids
   - regular exercise

9   Training and Retraining Bowels

- toileting client at regular intervals
- praise by aide at slightest progress of client
- less reliance on laxatives and enemas
- privacy for client during bowel movements

3. Follow bowel retraining program developed by the health care team. If plan appears to be working, note success of program. If plan does not work, report that fact. It is also important to give some suggestions to the health care team of possible solutions for retraining the client.

CLIENT CARE PROCEDURE

10   Insertion of a Rectal Suppository

PURPOSE

- To relieve a client of constipation
- To make the client more comfortable

NOTE: A rectal suppository is a cone-shaped, easily melted, medicated mass that can readily be inserted into a client's rectum. Suppositories are usually stored in the client's refrigerator and are wrapped in foil. The suppository will melt once inserted into the warm environment of the rectum and colon. The suppository contains ingredients that once absorbed by the lining of the colon will give a stimulus to the colon to evacuate stool. It takes the suppository at least five to ten minutes to melt. It is important that the aide inform the client to wait a few minutes after the suppository is inserted before trying to have a bowel movement.

PROCEDURE

1. Assemble supplies:
   - rectal suppository
   - gloves
   - lubricant
   - protective pad or paper towels
2. Wash hands and apply gloves.
3. Tell client what you plan to do.
4. Open foil-wrapped suppository. Turn client on one side.
5. Lubricate gloved finger and insert suppository into rectum (see Figure 6–32). Push the suppository along the lining of the rectum with your index finger as far as your finger allows. Be careful not to insert suppository into the feces. The suppository needs to be next to the lining of the colon for it to be effective.

10   Inserting of a Rectal Suppository

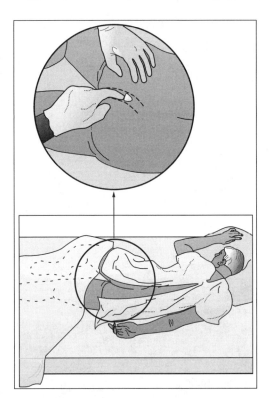

Figure 6–32 Carefully place the rectal suppository into the rectum about three inches on adult clients.

6. After ten minutes has passed, assist the client to the toilet or commode.
7. After client has had a bowel movement, assist client back to bed or chair.
8. Observe results of elimination.
9. Remove gloves and wash hands.
10. Record results. It is important to note color, consistency, and amount.

CLIENT CARE PROCEDURE

11   Administering a Commercial Enema

PURPOSE

- To relieve the client of constipation
- To prepare client for diagnostic tests
- To make the client more comfortable

NOTE: An enema is the introduction of fluid into the rectum to remove feces and flatus (gas) from the rectum and colon.

Because enemas distend or dilate the rectum, the client may experience a feeling of urgency in the bowel; that is, a very strong need to empty the bowel as soon as possible.

CLIENT CARE PROCEDURE , *continued*

11   Administering a Commercial Enema

Enemas can only be given on a doctor's orders.

The two commercially prepared enemas are the chemical (often referred to as Fleet®) and the oil-retention enemas. Oil retention enemas are given to soften hard feces in the rectum and are usually followed by a soap solution enema.

PROCEDURE

1. Assemble supplies (see Figure 6–33)
   - gloves
   - commercial prepackaged enema
   - protective pad
   - bedpan (if client is bedridden)
   - toilet paper
   - lubrication jelly

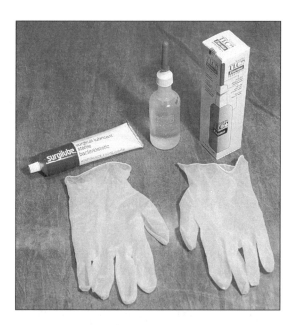

Figure 6–33   Equipment needed to administer a commercial enema

2. Wash hands and put on gloves.
3. Tell client what you plan to do.
4. Provide for the client's comfort and privacy.
5. Have client turn to left side. Turn covers back to expose only the buttocks.
6. Remove cover on tip of enema. Apply extra lubricant to tip to ensure easy insertion.
7. Place protective pad underneath the client's buttocks.
8. Separate the buttocks and insert tip into rectum at least three inches. Tell client to take a deep breath and hold the solution as long as possible. Slowly squeeze the flexible plastic tube (see Figure 6–34). This forces the solution to flow evenly into the rectum.
9. Remove enema tip while holding the client's buttocks together.

CLIENT CARE PROCEDURE, *continued*

11   Administering a Commercial Enema

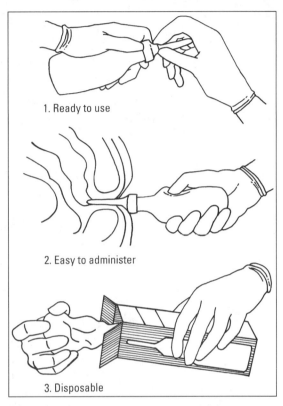

1. Ready to use

2. Easy to administer

3. Disposable

Figure 6–34 Administering a commercial enema. (Used with permission from C. B. Fleet Company, Inc., Lynchburg, VA)

10. Position client on bedpan, commode, or toilet.

11. After client has expelled feces and enema solution, assist the client in cleaning area around anus and buttocks.

12. Return client to comfortable position. It may be necessary to leave the protective pad in place until the effects of the enema are complete.

13. Remove gloves and wash hands.

14. Record results of enema as to color, amount, and consistency (for example, 10:00 AM, Fleet® enema given, good results, large, brown, formed stool).

Some areas on which to focus in bowel training are:

1. Observe the bowel pattern by keeping a record of the time and character of each bowel movement.

2. Have the nurse check for fecal impaction.

3. Observe for signs of constipation or diarrhea.

4. Report any abdominal or rectal discomfort.

5. Establish regularity by offering the bedpan or bedside commode at regular times.

Helpful Hints: Be careful not to communicate nonverbal messages, particularly facial expressions of disgust.

6. Administer bowel aides such as suppositories or laxatives as prescribed by the physician.

7. Offer a comfortable and private environment for the client to move their bowels.

8. If the client is unsuccessful, offer a warm drink to stimulate the bowel movement.

Adequate fluid intake is an important part of bowel training and to prevent constipation. Sometimes a special diet with increased fiber can be ordered by the physician to correct constipation. These diets encourage fresh, raw and cooked vegetables, and fruits, juices, whole grain products, protein-rich foods, bran and bran products, and good amounts of water. Bowel training can take up to eight weeks for a client and consistent support from the HCA, the health care team, and the family is important.

bladder training training to restore the client's ability to control urination

Bladder training is most often ordered for clients who have problems with retention of urine resulting in incontinence. Retraining the bladder takes from six to eight weeks and emotional support is a big factor in success. All members of the team, the client, and the family need to know what the training program involves and how to play a role in it. Figure 6–35 shows an example of a bladder retraining (as well as a bowel retraining) assessment. The client's understanding, participation, and cooperation are vital to the success of the program. Refer to Client Care Procedure 12 for retraining the bladder.

CLIENT CARE PROCEDURE

12   Retraining the Bladder

PURPOSE

- To regain bladder control

PROCEDURE

A home heath aide must keep a record of how often and how much the client voids throughout the day and night for a few days. Once the client's voiding pattern is known, the nurse/supervisor can analyze the client's voiding record and formulate a schedule for the aide to follow. The schedule developed by the nurse will include regularly scheduled times for the aide to have the client drink a measured amount of fluid. After the client has drunk the liquid, the aide notes the time. Thirty minutes later, the aide toilets the client. The aide should encourage the client to void each time he or she is positioned on the commode or toilet. It is helpful at times to run water from the faucet to give the client an urge to void. Other methods include having the client apply light pressure to the bladder area to stimulate the urge to empty the bladder or having the client lean forward on the toilet to stimulate emptying the bladder. Remember that the client needs to be toileted at regular intervals to prevent accidents. The client needs consistent positive reinforcement to remain dry. At first it may be necessary to take the client to the bathroom every two hours; intervals may be lengthened as control is gained. A common cause of incontinence is delay in getting

Comp. # 1983 Page 1, Film 1, One Color, Punches on Left

BLADDER RETRAINING ASSESSMENT
(Reference tags: F315, F316)

CURRENT CLIENT STATUS

DIAGNOSIS_____ **RESIDENT'S AGE**_____

RECENT SURGERY? ☐ Yes ☐ No If Yes, date ____/____/____ and type_____

CURRENT MEDICATIONS (i.e., Diuretics, Psychotropics, etc.)_____

_____

_____

Mental Status and Ability to Communicate	Mobility Status	Vision Status	Right	Left
☐ Alert	☐ Independent	Adequate	☐	☐
☐ Aphasic	☐ Transfer/standing ability	Adequate w/aid	☐	☐
☐ Oriented x_____	☐ Wheelchair bound	Poor	☐	☐
☐ Disoriented	☐ Bed rest	Blind	☐	☐
☐ Depressed	☐ Contractures			
☐ Cooperative	☐ Other_____	**Hearing Status**	**Right**	**Left**
☐ Uncooperative	_____	Adequate	☐	☐
☐ Slow comprehension	_____	Adequate w/aid	☐	☐
☐ Other_____	_____	Poor	☐	☐
	_____	Deaf	☐	☐

BLADDER ASSESSMENT

1. **LENGTH OF INCONTINENCE:** _____ Days _____ Months _____ Years

2. **REASON FOR INCONTINENCE (if known):** _____
   CATHETER: ☐ Yes ☐ No If Yes, specify type and size _____
   Date inserted ____/____/____ Reason for catheter _____

3. **USUAL VOIDING PATTERN:** Frequency _____ Amt./voiding _____ cc: /24 hrs. _____ cc
   Pattern: ☐ Upon arising ☐ After meals ☐ No apparent pattern ☐ Night time only
   ☐ Other (specify) _____

4. **SYMPTOMS:** (Check all that apply)
   ☐ Voids often in small amounts ☐ Difficulty stopping stream ☐ Urgency
   ☐ Fills bladder/voids large amount ☐ Dribbles constantly ☐ Burning/Pain
   ☐ Unable to void ☐ Dribbles after voiding ☐ Edema
   ☐ Difficulty starting stream ☐ Dribbles while coughing ☐ Other (specify)_____

5. **HISTORY OF:** ☐ Urinary Disorders ☐ Bladder Disorders ☐ Kidney Disease ☐ Prostate Problems
   ☐ Neurological Disorders ☐ Fecal Impactions ☐ Other (specify)_____

6. **RELIEF AFTER VOIDING:** ☐ Complete ☐ Continued desire to void

7. **BLADDER DISTENDED:** ☐ Yes ☐ No **EMPTIED BY EXTERNAL STIMULI:** ☐ Yes ☐ No
   If Yes, Check: ☐ Kegel Exercises ☐ Warm water over perineum
   ☐ Other (specify) _____

8. **RESIDUAL URINE:** ☐ Yes ☐ No If Yes, Amount: _____ cc

9. **PERCEPTION OF NEED TO VOID:** ☐ Present ☐ Diminished ☐ Absent

10. **WELL HYDRATED:** ☐ Yes ☐ No **AVERAGE FLUID INTAKE (24 HRS)** _____ cc
    AVERAGE FLUID OUTPUT (24 HRS) _____ cc
    Fluids Preferred _____

NAME—Last	First	Middle	Attending Physician	Chart No.

CFS 6-10HH © 1992 Briggs Corporation, Des Moines, IA 50306 (800) 247-2343 Printed in U.S.A.

BLADDER RETRAINING ASSESSMENT
☐ Continued on Reverse

Figure 6–35 Bladder retraining assessment sheet *(continues)*

Comp.#1983 Page 2, Film 1, One Color, Backer for HH

EVALUATION FOR BLADDER RETRAINING POTENTIAL

☐ ABLE TO PARTICIPATE IN RETRAINING   EVALUATION PERIOD: _____ TO _____

PLAN: _____

_____

PROVIDE FLUIDS:	FLUIDS SHOULD BE SPACED AS FOLLOWS:				
_____ cc every 24 Hrs	☐7AM	☐11	☐3PM	☐7	☐11PM ☐3
_____ cc 7-3 shift	☐8	☐12N	☐4	☐8	☐12MN ☐4
_____ cc 3-11 shift	☐9	☐1PM	☐5	☐9	☐1AM ☐5
_____ cc 11-7 shift	☐10	☐2	☐6	☐10	☐2 ☐6

OFFER NO FLUIDS AFTER ____ PM   TOILET FOR VOIDING EVERY ___ Hrs (Day and Evening) ___ Hrs (Night)
(Except as needed for medications)

RECORD RESULTS ON BLADDER RETRAINING RECORD. _____

☐ UNABLE TO PARTICIPATE IN RETRAINING

REASON: _____

_____

REEVALUATION DATE: _____

COMPLETED BY: _____   ___/___/___
Signature/Title   Date

BLADDER RETRAINING PROGRESS NOTES OR REEVALUATION NOTES

DATE	TIME	NOTES - ALL ENTRIES MUST BE SIGNED WITH NAME AND TITLE

NAME—Last	First	Middle	Attending Physician	Chart No.

BLADDER RETRAINING NOTES

Figure 6–35, *continued*

the client to the bathroom. It is of utmost importance to take the client to the bathroom on a regular time schedule. The plan also calls for the aide to maintain the client's fluid intake at about 2500 cc/day. The aide should encourage the client to wear regular underwear to enhance the client's self-esteem and to help him or her from reverting back to the previous incontinence habit.

Some of the areas to focus on in bladder retraining are:

1. Fluids should be encouraged during the daytime hours and restricted at night.
2. When offering the bedpan or commode, the client's positioning is important. Changing the height of the seat and handrails can offer increased comfort to the client. Men find it easier to urinate in a standing position.
3. Additional stimuli can encourage voiding (urinating) such as offering a glass of water, pouring water over the perineum, running water in the sink, bearing down to empty the bladder (unless contraindicated by the physician), and placing the client's hand in water.

Helpful Hints: Patience is the key to motivating the client in bowel and bladder training.

4. The skin should be thoroughly cleaned on the incontinent client on a regular basis.
5. Caregivers should offer to assist the client to urinate on a regular schedule (every three to four hours).
6. Keep a careful record of the time and amount of urination on the intake and output sheets. Include any special problem areas and successful techniques for this client so other caregivers can offer consistent care. Refer to Client Care Procedure 13 for recording intake and output.

CLIENT CARE PROCEDURE

13   Measuring and Recording Fluid Intake and Output

PURPOSE

- To identify food items that need to be measured for fluid intake
- To measure and record fluid intake and output accurately

NOTE: Intake is a measure of all the fluids or semiliquids that a person drinks. Output is all the fluid that passes out of the body. The abbreviation for measuring fluid intake and output is I&O. Figure 6–36 shows the fluids that should be included in the measurement of intake and output.

PROCEDURE

1. Assemble supplies.
   - measuring cup or container for intake
   - large measuring container for output

13 Measuring and Recording Fluid Intake and Output

PROCEDURE

Measure for Intake

ice	water
juices	pop
coffee	ice cream
yogurt	soup
Jell-o®	pudding
any other food that is liquid at room temperature	

Measure for Output

vomitus (emesis)	liquid stools
urine	
blood or drainage from wounds	

Figure 6–36 Various fluids and substances are measured and recorded as intake and output.

2. Wash hands and apply gloves if measuring output.

3. Measure and record all liquids taken by the client. This includes all fluids taken with meals and between meals such as coffee, milk, fruit juices, beer, and water. Liquids are recorded in cubic centimeters, abbreviated cc (see Figure 6–37). Remember that 30 cc equals 1 ounce, so if a client drank a can of pop that was 12 ounces, multiple 12 by 30 to equal 360 cc.

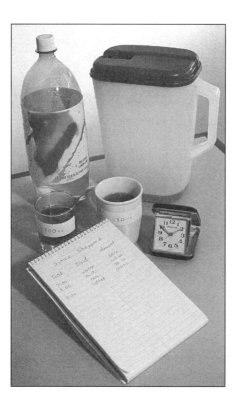

Figure 6–37 Measure the cubic centimeter (cc) capacity of commonly used glasses and cups. Record intake in cubic centimeters (cc) after the client has drunk the fluid.

13 Measuring and Recording Fluid Intake and Output

4. Ask the client to use a urinal or bedpan for all voiding. If the client can use the toilet, a special plastic "hat" can be placed in the toilet to collect the urine (see Figure 6–38). All urine must be collected so that it can be measured.

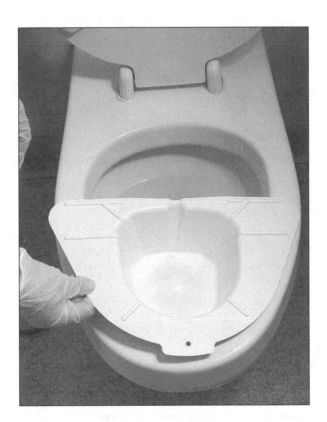

Figure 6–38 If a client's urine needs to be measured, a special toilet insert (potty hat) may be used to collect it.

5. Pour urine from bedpan or urinal into a measuring device (see Figure 6–39). Record the amount. Always record output in cc.

13 Measuring and Recording Fluid Intake and Output

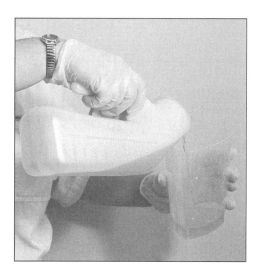

Figure 6–39 Urine can be measured with a special plastic container or a large measuring cup.

6. Be sure to explain to the client how to keep exact records. The client must record the fluids at times when the aide is off duty.
7. Clean equipment after each use.
8. Remove gloves and wash hands.

PERSONAL CARE

Personal care procedures for rehabilitation clients are offered to assist them in returning to self-care. It is important that the client feels that progress is being made during this long rehabilitation period. Often, providing their own personal care in small stages is the only real progress clients feel is occurring. Some of the reasons that rehabilitation clients cannot perform personal care for themselves might be:

- weakness of the arms and shoulders
- inability to remember the sequence of tasks
- poor judgment
- inability to remember items and their use for personal care
- depression
- indifference to appearance

Some of the personal care activities with which disabled clients have problems are:

- bathing
- shaving
- mouth and denture care
- hair care
- skin care
- nail care
- foot care
- perineal care
- feeding
- applying toiletries (make-up or after-shave lotion)

When assisting the client with personal care, the HCA must have patience and explain to the client slowly and carefully what is to be done. The occupational therapist or nurse will probably develop techniques for the disabled client and caregivers to follow. The following are some guidelines for assisting functionally limited persons with personal care:

1. Do not begin to assist the client before he or she is ready, both physically and emotionally.
2. Follow the plan developed by the OT or the nurse.
3. Provide a safe and healthy environment for the client.
4. Assemble and place all equipment where the client can reach it easily.
5. Remind the client of areas he or she may forget.
6. Always wash the involved arm or leg first.
7. Demonstrate proper techniques such as rinsing and patting dry.
8. Assist the client with controlling the temperature of water.
9. Offer to do the personal care areas the client cannot reach or do easily.
10. Never rush or ridicule the client.

Always use the time with the client for observing the client's body and condition.

HOME MAINTENANCE

home maintenance keeping the home as a safe and healthy environment

A duty the HCA might have to provide in the home of the client needing rehabilitation is **home maintenance**. If the caretaker of the home is the client, other members of the family may not be familiar with caring for the home. The role the HCA plays in maintaining a healthy and clean environment for the client usually includes light housekeeping, laundry, shopping, and meal service.

A clean home offers fewer risks of infection and accidents and promotes a comfortable surrounding for the client. Many times, home maintenance duties involve the client's bedroom, the kitchen, and bathroom areas. If the HCA is not in the home for long periods of time, it is important to set up a schedule with other team members and caregivers so that household tasks can be distributed. The following are some important areas to remember in home maintenance:

1. Keep the home organized and tidy.
2. Keep a shopping list so that cleaning supplies and laundry items are available.
3. Keep kitchen floors clean from spills and crumbs.
4. Air the client's room (if weather permits) to reduce the risk of infection.
5. Store food properly in the kitchen.
6. Check the cupboards for food and keep a shopping list up to date.
7. Keep the bathroom clean at all times to avoid the spread of microorganisms.
8. Clean the tubs, sinks, and shower every day.
9. Keep bathroom floors free of spills to avoid accidents.
10. Delegate someone in the family to keep a good supply of linens on hand for the client's daily use.

AMPUTATION OF LOWER EXTREMITIES

amputation the surgical removal of all or part of a limb, usually one of the lower extremities, above or below the knee

The surgical removal of all or part of a limb, usually the lower extremity above or below the knee, is called **amputation**. Causes for amputation include:

- serious circulatory problems
- uncontrollable infections
- gangrene (tissue death)
- severe trauma
- cancer

The HCA who cares for a client after a recent amputation of a lower extremity may be required to provide care to the stump. There are important considerations related to a recent amputation of an extremity with which the HCA should be familiar. These include:

- observing the surgical site for increased redness, swelling, or signs of infection.
- observing the stump for poor circulation evidenced by coldness of the skin and/or poor healing.
- observing the stump for excessive bleeding or drainage.
- observing the client for pain and discomfort.

Care of the client with an amputation also includes careful observation for signs of complications such as:

- phantom limb pain in which clients experience pain or tingling where the limb used to be. This may occur for up to a month after surgery and is caused by spasms of the muscles.
- contracture deformities
- mental depression or grieving for the loss of the body part.
- loss of self-esteem.
- pressure sores resulting from the difference in weight-bearing with the amputated extremity, improper wrapping of the stump, or an improper fit of the prosthesis.

To prevent hip and knee contractures, the following positioning guidelines are valuable:

- Never place pillows under the stump. Maintain the stump flat on the bed with the knee extended.
- Maintain the hips flat on the bed.
- Keep legs abducted.
- Avoid long periods of the client sitting and standing.
  Care of the stump includes the following:
- Washing with mild soap and water, drying gently, and allowing to air dry well before wrapping.
- Avoiding powders and creams which irritate and soften the skin.
- Providing good skin care.
- Wrapping the stump with a stump sock, an elastic bandage, or a stump shrinker if ordered by the physician. Avoid wrapping the stump too tightly and rewrap at least twice daily.

When the client is fitted with a prosthesis, the HCA should provide the following care and support:

- Assist the client to apply the prosthesis after the nurse or PT has instructed the client and family on how to properly attach it.

- Assist in ambulation as ordered by the nurse or physician.
- Report any changes in skin condition such as blisters, rashes, or pressure sores.
- Provide assistance to the client for safe transfer techniques and client self-care of the stump.
- Maintain a clean, healthy, and safe environment, free from danger of falls because these clients have poor balance.
- Provide adequate fluids and nutrition.

The PT will fit the prosthesis and teach the client how to use it. Some home exercises may be ordered to strengthen muscles, promote circulation, decrease edema, and decrease shrinkage of the stump. Early in the rehabilitation program, the client may use crutches or a wheelchair. The PT or the physician will determine when it is safe for the client to begin walking.

REVIEW QUESTIONS

1. List the five basic gaits.
   a.
   b.
   c.
   d.
   e.
2. List the three benefits of ROM exercises.
   a.
   b.
   c.
3. _____ _____ are used to prevent the client's hips and legs from turning outward when he or she is lying in bed.
4. List four supportive devices for positioning clients.
   a.
   b.
   c.
   d.
5. True or False? ROMs are always done by the HCA
6. True or False? One or more pillows are frequently useful when repositioning the client.
7. True or False? Maintaining the home as a clean and safe environment is a role of the HCA.
8. True or False? Proper skin care can help prevent decubitus ulcers.
9. Unscramble the following key term from the chapter: mheo atnmannceie _____

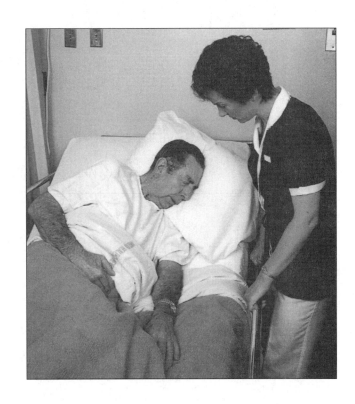

CHAPTER 7

Pain Reduction and Control

OBJECTIVES

Upon reading this chapter and completing the review questions, the home care aide should be able to:

1. Recognize the important techniques involved in pain management.
2. Define the role of the TENS unit for pain relief.
3. Describe aspects of joint and hip pain and the HCA's role.

KEY TERMS

distractions   TENS unit

hip disorders   weight-bearing

pain management

INTRODUCTION

Because clients requiring rehabilitation frequently have pain and discomfort, it is vital that the HCA be aware of pain control and reduction methods. This chapter discusses various disease conditions and methods of keeping the client as comfortable as possible.

PAIN MANAGEMENT

pain management   pain control through techniques to reduce discomfort

Pain management involves pain control through various techniques to reduce the client's discomfort. It is important that the client's pain level be kept at a minimum so that the rehabilitation process can be performed in a comfortable manner. There are many techniques available to reduce pain for clients with musculoskeletal problems. Clients are more apt to perform their PT, OT, or ST exercises if they are comfortable. Arthritis and joint disabilities are especially painful. The following are types of pain control techniques with which the HCA, with a written plan of care, might assist:

- prescribed medications
- heat applications
- heated pool, tub, or shower
- rest periods
- massage
- stress management
- braces
- relaxation techniques
- cold applications
- strengthening exercises
- stretching exercises
- the TENS unit
- distractions
- music therapy
- energy conservation
- assistive devices
- a walk

Pain management techniques can be incorporated by the HCA following the daily plan of care. A positive attitude and words of encouragement are more valuable than sympathy for clients with chronic pain problems. The HCA can be important in the observation and reporting phases of pain management by being careful to note the location of the pain, the degree of the pain (on a scale from one to ten with ten being the most severe), how long the pain lasts, when the pain started, and what if anything relieves the pain. The HCA should also observe the client's body language for symptoms of pain (see Figure 7–1).

If clients are on pain medication, it is important to observe the frequency of the use of the medication as well as its effects. Abuse of medications for relief of pain is common in the chronically disabled. Overuse of medications can lead to accidents and

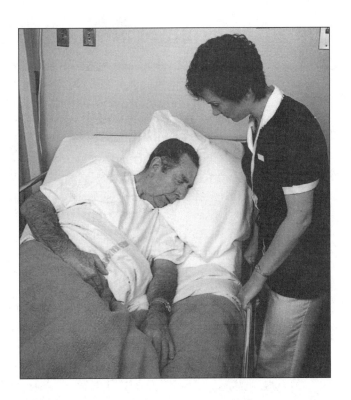

Figure 7–1 Sometimes the client who is experiencing pain reveals this information through body language.

TENS unit electrical stimulation of nerves to reduce pain

distractions activities or techniques to change the client's focus from his or her pain

Helpful Hints: The HCA and caregiver may be very creative in finding just the right distraction for each client.

falls as well as mental and emotional problems. Encouragement and some of the other treatments mentioned above can be used in addition to, or in place of, pain medication.

The **TENS unit** is sometimes ordered by the physician as a means of pain relief and works with electrical stimulation of nerve fibers in the skin. It can be used in the home by the PT in addition to vibration, heat, cold, topical creams, and massage. A TENS unit is applied to the skin. It runs on a battery and creates a tingling sensation in the area of pain. Frequently, the TENS unit is used with local applications of cold to the painful area. It has been discovered that cold does not necessarily cause muscles to contract but can, in short applications, cause muscle relaxation and is, therefore, applied for pain relief with or without the TENS unit. The client can wear a TENS unit twenty-four hours a day. If the HCA does not understand how it functions, the PT or the nurse should be consulted for instructions. The HCA may assist the patient to apply the TENS electrodes if instructed to do so on the plan of care.

One of the most effective techniques for pain relief is **distractions** which increase the client's tolerance for pain. Music therapy and relaxation techniques are two methods of distraction. Meditation is sometimes effective, and offering a quiet environment may lower the client's pain threshold. Watching television and listening to the radio are simple distraction techniques. Deep breathing exercises can be helpful as well as guided imagery in which the client relaxes and a caregiver takes him or her on an imagined journey to a beautiful place.

HIP JOINT PAIN

hip disorders   disease or injury to the hip such as arthritis, fractures, dislocation, and hip surgery

Clients with **hip disorders** are commonly seen in home health-care situations and the HCA should be familiar with some of the problems associated with caring for clients with hip injuries. Early discharge from hospitals for clients with hip fractures and hip surgery creates increasing case loads for the home health industry. Clients commonly stay in the hospital for several days during which time ambulation and physical therapy are usually begun. There are 120,000 hips replaced in the United States every year and the success of such surgery is well documented. However, it is up to the home care team to see that the client progresses with the normal rehabilitation in the follow-up care that is offered in the home. Physical therapy is very important and the physician will order what therapies are safe for the client. The goal is to have the client return to walking at as normal a level as possible. Usually, the client begins with variations in **weight-bearing**, from no weight-bearing (NWB) to partial weight-bearing (PWB) using crutches or a walker, and eventually to full weight-bearing (FWB) or being able to walk with the use of a cane or without any assistive devices.

weight-bearing   amount of body weight placed on a hip or leg

Clients who have hip fractures must never rotate the affected leg outward. The knee always should be kept below the hips and the client should not bend more than 90 degrees from the waist. A pillow between the legs can support the affected leg to keep it away from the midline of the body (abduction). The alignment of this leg is important as well as orders from the physician concerning weight-bearing and posture when ambulating.

Some special guidelines to remember for clients with hip fractures are:

- never permit the client to lie on his or her side with legs together (touching)
- never rotate or turn the affected leg outward
- never allow the client to bend forward from the waist to pull up socks or tie shoes (use adaptive equipment)
- always use a high chair and do not allow the client to cross his or her legs or raise the knee

Helpful Hints: The HCA should always check with the supervisor or the nurse to see what movements the client is permitted.

After hip surgery, therapeutic exercises are supervised by the PT to increase ambulation and function. It is especially important that the physician write an order for the degree of weight-bearing that the client is permitted. Ambulatory assistive devices must be used with caution because these clients are at greater risk for injury from falls.

The HCA might assist the nurse caring for the client with hip fractures or hip surgery with the following:

- observing the wound for signs of infection
- observing the family in safety of transfers and ambulation
- observing the client's medication program
- providing personal care
- maintaining nutrition
- maintaining the home
- positioning and exercising the affected hip as determined by the type of correction or surgery done

Pain may be more obvious when the client is having physical therapy or after physical therapy and the HCA should encourage the client to rest after therapy. In addition, the family could offer periods of attention and amusement at that vital time of the day.

REVIEW QUESTIONS

1. List five examples of pain control techniques.

   a.

   b.

   c.

   d.

   e.

2. On a scale of one to ten, the most severe pain is described as number _____ .

3. Name four HCA duties for patients with hip surgery.

   a.

   b.

   c.

   d.

4. True or False? Watching television and listening to music can provide pain relief.

5. True or False? The nurse can determine the amount of weight-bearing the patient may perform.

6. True or False? Overuse of pain medications can lead to accidents and mental problems.

7. True or False? TENS units are ordered for relief of pain.

8. Unscramble the following key term from the chapter: anpi nammetngea _____ _____

8

Client/Family Education

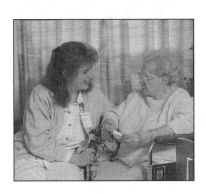

OBJECTIVES

Upon reading this chapter and completing the review questions, the home care aide should be able to:

1. Recognize the nurse's educational plan and factors for success.
2. Motivate and encourage the client and his or her family to respond to the teaching.
3. Understand the educational process and the HCA's role.

KEY TERMS

compliance	empower
educational plan	motivation

INTRODUCTION

In the home health arena, it is vital that the rehabilitation process be a team effort. In Chapter 4, we determined the multidisciplinary team. The home health care team consists of all trained personnel involved in the client's day-to-day care and treatment. There are two other members of the team who play the greatest part in the success or failure of the recuperation of the client. These are the client and the client's family. Very few rehabilitation programs would last without the full cooperation and participation of the client and his or her family. This is accomplished through a comprehensive educational plan.

THE EDUCATIONAL PLAN

education plan   the day-to-day organization and process of the client/family teaching procedure prepared by the nurse

It is important for the HCA to understand the **educational plan** and to keep current on its progress or lack of progress. Also, the HCA who specializes in caring for clients requiring rehabilitation must accept a responsibility to meet the following four main goals of client/family education:

- Always have a clear understanding of the client's day-to-day condition and how that is reflected in the documentation and HCA and nursing care plans.

- Observe and report any family needs, questions, or problems to the supervisor by keeping channels of communication open at all times.

- Know and understand which educational and teaching methods the therapist and/or nurse assigned to the case are using for the client/family so there will be consistent follow-up to their instructions.

- Act as a professional role model and set a good example to the client/family as procedures and tasks are performed from day to day.

Helpful Hints: Keep the client's educational materials in a special "Home Care Corner" so all members of the team and the family have easy access to them.

Because the health care team cannot be in the home twenty-four hours a day, the recovery process must be continued by the family. For this reason, the education provided to give the client and family the knowledge and skills to continue the care is important. The ultimate goal of home health care is to return the client to the highest level of function. Without proper education, this is not possible.

One of the most important skills the nurse uses in home health nursing is teaching and training the client and family. Medicare and other payors for rehabilitation care recognize the importance of education and consider it a reasonable expense. The nurse on the case will develop a teaching plan based on:

- the physician's orders
- the client/family role
- the condition of the client
- the number of visits covered
- the nursing and HCA care plans
- the long-term and short-term client goals
- the expected outcome

Factors to consider in the success of client/family education include:

- the severity of the illness
- ages of the learners

compliance how well the client/family responds to the educational process

motivation to encourage another person to action

- education level of the learners
- mental status of the learners
- **compliance**
- **motivation**
- understanding the importance of education
- understanding the importance of goals

The HCA's role in the education process is to:

- offer follow-up teaching if appropriate
- serve as a role model and good example
- interact and observe the level of the client and family's ability and learning

Some examples of follow-up teaching the HCA might do include:

- observe nutrition, fluid intake, and diet education taught by the dietitian
- observe exercises taught by the therapist or nurse
- observe speech and occupational exercises taught by the therapists

Situations in which the HCA would serve as a role model might include:

- motivating the client/family
- utilizing infection control practices
- offering a positive and encouraging manner
- practicing good personal hygiene
- displaying a patient and caring attitude (see Figure 8-1)

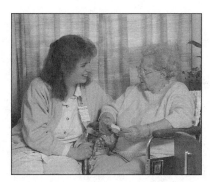

Figure 8–1 Positive reinforcement such as praise encourages and motivates the client.

- observing the client while performing personal care
- performing procedures well
- following good safety rules
- showing respect for the client's home
- being dependable and courteous

Some situations in which the HCA will have opportunities to interact with and observe the client and family's abilities and level of learning include:

- client verbal communication during ADLs
- family verbal communication during visit
- client nonverbal communication behavior during personal care
- family nonverbal communication behavior during visit
- involving both family and client in reviewing the care plan.

During the educational sessions, it is important to remember:

- the environment should be comfortable and quiet with no distractions such as television, radio, or visitors.
- the educational materials should be interesting and at the learner's level of understanding.
- the teacher should speak slowly and clearly and demonstrate patience by repeating when necessary.
- positive reinforcement such as praise instead of criticism encourages learning
- the educational period should be short, organized, and convenient to the learner
- the educational content should be taught in a step-by-step plan
- the teacher should demonstrate by example and not rush through a session

empower   to authorize or strongly encourage another person

The final result of good client and family education is to **empower** these persons to reach their highest potential. The areas most often addressed in home health care in rehabilitation education are:

- ambulation and exercise with or without assistive devices
- self-care of personal needs such as bathing, skin care, hair and nail care, and mouth care
- waste elimination from bladder and bowel including fluid changes
- self-administration of medications
- understanding disease or injury condition and preventing complications
- safety measures
- infection control practices
- care and use of equipment
- nutrition, diet, preparation of food, and self-feeding
- speech and motor skills

REVIEW QUESTIONS

1. Give examples of the four main goals of client/family education:

    a. An example of documentation that reflects the client's condition is using _____ .

    b. Some observable and reportable family problems might be _____ nutrition.

    c. A method of teaching that a therapist or nurse might use that the HCA should understand is _____ .

    d. An example of the HCA as a role model might be a _____ attitude.

2. List four factors that affect the teaching plan.

    a.

    b.

    c.

    d.

3. Name two situations in which the HCA can interact with the family and observe their levels of learning.

    a.

    b.

4. True or False? Comfort in the environment is important in the learning process of the client/family.

5. True or False? The nurse or therapist will teach infection control measures, but the HCA will serve as a good or bad example.

6. Unscramble the following key term from the chapter: natvoimiot _____

CHAPTER 9

SAFETY AND EMERGENCIES

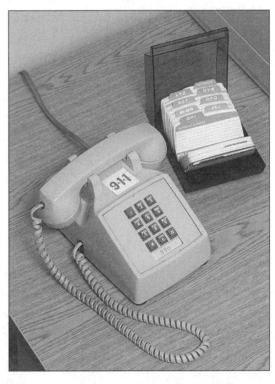

OBJECTIVES

Upon reading this chapter and completing the review questions, the home care aide should be able to:

1. Have a greater understanding of safety and emergency situations.
2. Observe the environment of the client in terms of safety measures.
3. Name the most common safety hazards in the home.
4. List some conditions that promote safety and prevent falls.
5. State some basic facts of medication safety.
6. Be familiar with emergency measures in home care.
7. Demonstrate an understanding of positioning the client and transfer safety.

KEY TERMS

aseptic

confused

disoriented

flammable

infection

pathogens

personal protective equipment (PPE)

safe environment

standard precautions

INTRODUCTION

safe environment an environment in which a person has a very low risk of illness or injury

The home can be an unsafe area for the homebound client as well as for the HCA who cares for that client. Clients who are ill and weak are more prone to accidents at home and are usually unable to handle an emergency.

Safety is one of the HCA's responsibilities. He or she can create a **safe environment** for the client by preventing, correcting, or eliminating conditions that could cause accidents and assisting the client and family in taking measures to be prepared for crisis intervention.

MAINTAINING A SAFE ENVIRONMENT IN THE HOME

When the patient is admitted to home health care, the skilled nurse does a safety assessment of the home during the admission process. A safety checklist is usually included in the admission packet because safety measures and interventions will begin at that time. The HCA follows up on this process and the nurse includes the client's family and the rest of the health care team when setting safety goals and determining if the goals have been met. The HCA should constantly assess the quality of the environment and look for safety hazards. If any are discovered, the HCA should report them to the supervisor immediately.

A safe environment is one in which a person has a very low risk of illness or injury. Some elderly and frail persons cannot assume the responsibility for their own safety. Poor vision may play a part in a client's inability to be safe at home. This could lead to falls, tripping, and misreading labels. Hearing loss is another factor affecting the client's safety as warning signals, such as fire detectors, may or may not be heard.

Helpful Hints: The agency is responsible for the client's safety. Therefore, the HCA, as the agency's representative, is also responsible for the client's safety.

The most common safety hazards in the home are:

- damaged electrical wiring on large and small appliances
- faulty or uneven stairs
- loose rugs that slip or slide
- poisons

flammable able to catch fire

- **flammable** cleaning rags, mops, and brooms
- sharp objects such as knives, razors, and lawn tools
- wet floors
- cluttered hallways or stairs (see Figure 9–1)
- unstable furniture
- electrical cords that are faulty (see Figure 9–2A)
- too many appliances plugged into one outlet (see Figure 9–2B)

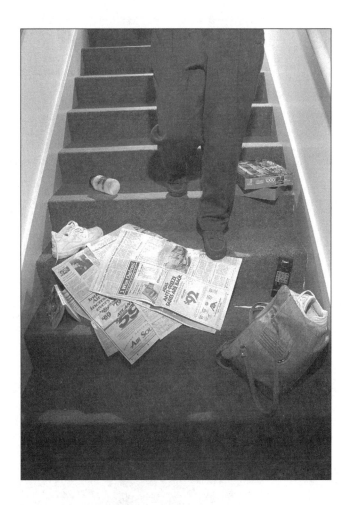

Figure 9–1 A cluttered stairway can be hazardous for the elderly client who has vision or balance problems.

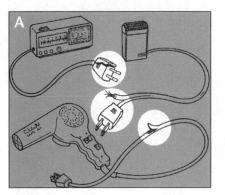

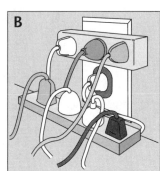

Figure 9–2 A. Cords in unsafe conditions. B. There are too many cords in this outlet.

Falls

Falls are the most common accidents in the home, particularly among the elderly. Most falls occur in the bedroom or bathroom and are caused by slippery floors, throw rugs, poor lighting, cluttered floors, furniture that is out of place, or slippery bathtubs and showers. Some conditions that promote safety and prevent falls are:

1. Adequate lighting which should be provided in rooms and hallways.

2. Hand rails on both sides of stairs, in halls, and in bathrooms (see Figure 9–3).

3. Carpeting that is tacked down and throw rugs discarded or put away.

4. Nonskid shoes and slippers worn by clients when ambulating.

5. Nonskid waxes on hardwood, tiled, or linoleum floors.

6. Floors uncluttered with toys and other objects.

7. Electrical cords and extension cords that are kept out of the path of the client.

8. Furniture must be left in place and not rearranged.

9. A telephone and lamp placed at the bedside.

10. Nonskid bathmats in tubs and showers.

11. Assisting clients when walking, getting out of bed, getting out of the tub or shower, and with other activities ordered by the physician.

12. A call bell within easy reach.

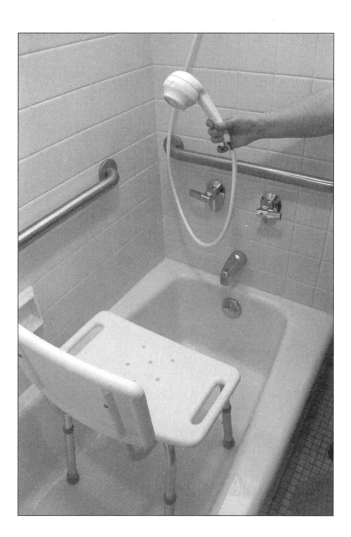

Figure 9–3 Safety features for the tub include several types of bars, nonskid strips, and bathing chair.

13. Cracked steps, loose hand rails, and frayed carpets reported and repaired promptly.

14. Frequently used items placed within the client's easy reach.

15. The client's bed in the low position, except when bedside care is being given to minimize the distance from the bed to the floor if the client falls or gets out of bed.

16. Nightlights in the client's room kept on at night.

17. Floors kept free of spills and excess furniture.

18. Crutches, canes, and walkers fitted with nonskid tips.

19. Wheels on beds and wheelchairs locked when transferring clients to or from them.

20. Gates at the tops and bottoms of stairs when there are infants and toddlers in the home. The child should not be able to put his or her head through the gate bars.

21. Side rails installed on the client's bed if possible to prevent him or her from falling out of bed.

MEDICATION SAFETY

Helpful Hints: Caregivers must keep their eyes and ears open for over-the-counter medication use and misuse that should be reported to the nurse and/or supervisor.

Storage and disposal of medications in the home are major problem areas for home health workers. HCAs should never dispense or administer medication. However, the HCA needs information about certain medications because many clients receiving home care services are taking them. HCAs often hand medications to their clients, remind clients to take medications, and report their use, misuse, and effects to their supervisors.

Some safety guidelines for medications include:

1. When cleaning the medicine cabinet, special care should be taken not to disturb medication container labels. The containers should be replaced in the same position in the medicine cabinet because often, clients expect a bottle to be in one position and do not look at the label.

2. If more than one person in the household is taking medications, keep the medications in separate rooms to avoid a client from taking the wrong medication.

3. Encourage the client to dispose of old medications correctly by flushing them down the toilet and report the disposal to the supervisor.

4. The client should store medications in a specific area and tell the family members where it is. The medications should not be moved.

5. Know if there are special instructions for storage of medications such as refrigeration.

6. Never refer to medications as candy.

The *five rights* for safely taking medications are:

1. The *right* client
2. The *right* medication
3. The *right* time
4. The *right* way to take the medication (oral, for example)
5. The *right* dose

EMERGENCY MEASURES IN HOME CARE

HCAs may be called upon to handle emergency situations in the home. All HCAs should have a basic first aid course and a current basic life support course.

Emergency Plans

Helpful Hints: All HCAs should keep current on CPR and emergency measures at all times.

Each emergency situation is different. The following rules apply to any kind of emergency:

1. HCAs should know their limitations and not attempt any procedure that is unfamiliar.
2. HCAs should remain calm at all times. Being calm helps the victim feel more secure.
3. HCAs should observe the client for life-threatening problems and should always check for breathing, pulse, and bleeding.
4. HCAs should keep the victim lying down or in the position in which he or she was found and should not move the victim. Moving a victim could make the injury worse.
5. HCAs should perform necessary emergency measures.
6. HCAs should call for help or instruct someone to call 911. An operator will then send emergency vehicles and personnel to the scene. The person calling 911 should give the following information to the operator:
   - The location including the street address and city or town.
   - The phone number where the victim is located.
   - What happened (a fall, choking, or the like) since fire equipment, police, or ambulances might be needed.
   - How many people require emergency medical attention.
   - The condition(s) of the victim(s), any obvious injuries, and if there is a life-threatening situation.
   - What aid if any, is currently being given.
7. HCAs should not remove any clothing unless absolutely necessary.

8. The victim should be kept warm. Aides can cover the victim with a blanket or a coat.

9. HCAs should reassure the conscious victim by explaining what is happening and that help is on the way.

10. HCAs should not give the victim any foods or fluids.

11. HCAs should keep onlookers away from the victim to maintain his or her privacy.

Every home should have a plan in case of emergencies (see Figure 9–4). The home with an elderly, frail, ill, or impaired person must take extra measures to plan ahead for emergency situations.

Reporting an accident or emergency by telephone should be done in a calm manner. It is important to have emergency numbers written down next to the telephone(s). Figure 9–5 shows an example of what numbers should be posted next to the telephone. This list should include:

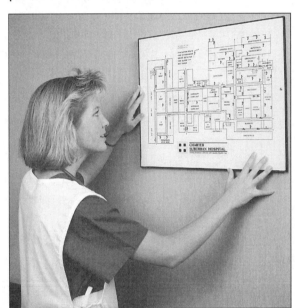

Figure 9–4 Client and family should know the escape plan in the event of a fire.

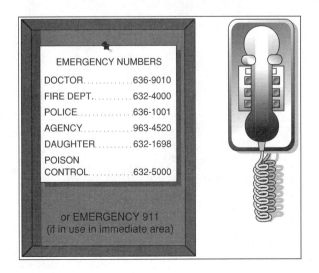

Figure 9–5 Important numbers should be posted by the telephone.

- Emergency Medical Services (EMS), often 911, if available
- Police department
- Fire department
- Responsible family member at work
- The home care supervisor and agency
- Client's physician
- Nearest hospital
- Ambulance service (if different from EMS)
- Poison control center

If there is no telephone in the client's home, arrange in advance to use a neighbor's telephone in case of an emergency.

FIRE SAFETY

There are three major causes of fires in this country: faulty electrical equipment and wiring, overloaded electrical circuits, and smoking. Figure 9–6 shows the elements needed for combustion. Fire safety measures include:

1. Following the fire safety precautions for the use of oxygen.
2. Making sure all ashes, cigar, and cigarette butts are out before emptying ashtrays.
3. Providing ashtrays to clients who are allowed to smoke.
4. Emptying ashtrays into a metal container partly filled with sand or water. Do not empty ashtrays into wastebaskets or plastic containers lined with paper or plastic bags.
5. Supervising smoking clients who cannot protect themselves. This includes **confused**, **disoriented**, and sedated clients.
6. Following the safety practices for using electrical equipment.
7. Supervising the play of children and keeping matches out of their reach.

confused　mentally uncertain or unclear

disoriented　confusion as to identity or location

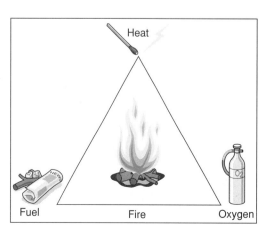

Figure 9–6　The fire triangle—elements needed for combustion (burning)

The following guidelines will help the HCA protect the client if there is a fire. The HCA should:

- have fire emergency numbers near the client's telephones
- call the fire department
- plan escape routes from each room
- know where fire extinguishers are and how to use them
- know where fire alarm boxes are located
- turn off any oxygen or electrical equipment in the general area of the fire
- get the client and others out of the house
- try to fight a small fire, if possible but leave right away if the fire gets out of control
- close door if the home is vacated
- crawl, keeping heads close to the floor if the area is filled with smoke
- cover faces with a damp cloth or towel in a smoke-filled area (see Figure 9–7)
- feel any doors before they are opened; do not open a door that feels hot or if smoke is coming from around the door
- open doors slowly, keeping the head to the side
- close doors immediately if smoke or heat rushes in

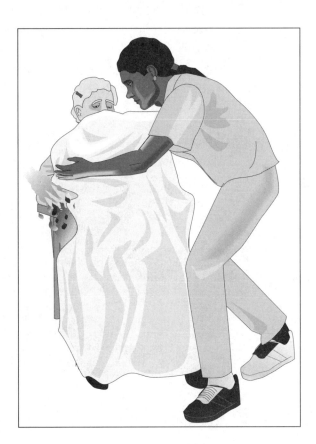

Figure 9–7 The HCA protects the client while trying to extinguish the fire.

- stuff blankets, clothes, towels, linens, coats, or other cloth along the bottom of the door if the client is trapped inside.

- Open window for air and hang a piece of cloth outside to attract attention.

The HCA should be able to use a fire extinguisher. Local fire departments often give demonstrations on how to operate a fire extinguisher and some agencies require all employees to demonstrate their use.

If an aide uses a fire extinguisher on a minor fire, the manufacturer's operating instructions must be carefully followed (see Figures 9–8A and B). Most extinguishers have a lock on the handle that must be unlocked before use. The extinguisher should be held firmly and the nozzle aimed at the near edge of the fire. Caution: Do not aim the nozzle toward the center of the fire. Discharge the extinguisher, using a slow, side-to-side motion, until the fire is out. Avoid contact with the chemical residues from the extinguisher. To prevent personal injury, always stay a safe distance from the fire.

An easy to remember method for operating a fire extinguisher is to follow the letters P-A-S-S:

P *Pull* the pin at the top of the extinguisher that keeps the handle from being pressed. Break the plastic or thin wire inspection band as the pin is pulled.

A *Aim* the nozzle or outlet toward the fire. Some hose assemblies are clipped to the extinguisher body. Release the hose and point.

S *Squeeze* the handle above the carrying handle to discharge the contents of the container. The handle can be released to

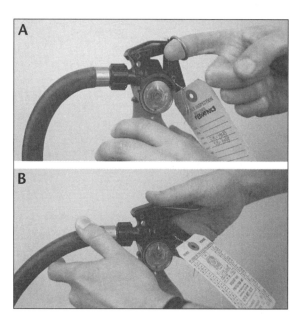

Figure 9–8 To use a fire extinguisher, (A) remove pin and (B) push top handle down.

stop the discharge at any time. Before approaching the fire, try a very short test burst to ensure proper operation.

S *Sweep* the nozzle back and forth at the base of the flames to disperse the extinguishing agent. After the fire is out, watch for remaining smoldering hot spots or possible reignition of flammable liquids. Make sure that the fire is out.

INFECTION CONTROL

infection germs entering the body and causing disease

All home health personnel must be careful to use proper measures to control **infection**. The client in a rehabilitation program is at no greater or lesser risk for infection than any other client. The specialized HCAs should keep current on the latest information to protect the client, the family, other workers, and themselves from infection.

Universal Precautions

pathogen disease-causing microorganism

Universal precautions were developed in 1985 by the Centers for Disease Control and Prevention (CDC). These guidelines were adhered to until they were updated in 1996. They are now called standard precautions. These guidelines apply to all health care workers concerning all clients, no matter what their diagnosis or where their care is given. If proper precautions are not taken, **pathogens** can be transmitted by the HCAs to clients, their families, other clients and their families, or even to the HCAs themselves by way of skin and clothing. Universal precautions protect against many different types of infections including AIDS, tuberculosis (TB), and Hepatitis B.

Standard Precautions

standard precautions guidelines published by the CDC to prevent the spread of pathogens to health care workers from their clients

The Centers for Disease Control and Prevention published new recommendations in 1996 called **standard precautions**. This new information is based on several years of research and data collection and helps to:

1. Improve the criteria for universal precautions.
2. Change some of the medical terminology.
3. Offer new information on drug resistant pathogens.
4. Update isolation guidelines.

Figure 9–9 illustrates the standard precautions.

STANDARD PRECAUTIONS FOR INFECTION CONTROL

Wash Hands (Plain soap)
Wash after touching blood, body fluids, secretions, excretions, and contaminated items. Wash immediately after gloves are removed and between patient contacts. Avoid transfer of microorganisms to other patients or environments.

Wear Gloves
Wear when touching blood, body fluids, secretions, excretions, and contaminated items. Put on clean gloves just before touching mucous membranes and nonintact skin. Change gloves between tasks and procedures on the same patient after contact with material that may contain high concentrations of microorganisms. Remove gloves promptly after use, before touching noncontaminated items and environmental surfaces, and before going to another patient, and wash hands immediately to avoid transfer of microorganisms to other patients or environments.

Wear Mask and Eye Protection or Face Shield
Protect mucous membranes of the eyes, nose and mouth during procedures and patient-care activities that are likely to generate splashes or sprays of blood, body fluids, secretions, or excretions.

Wear Gown
Protect skin and prevent soiling of clothing during procedures that are likely to generate splashes or sprays of blood, body fluids, secretions, or excretions. Remove a soiled gown as promptly as possible and wash hands to avoid transfer of microorganisms to other patients or environments.

Patient-Care Equipment
Handle used patient-care equipment soiled with blood, body fluids, secretions, or excretions in a manner that prevents skin and mucous membrane exposures, contamination of clothing, and transfer of microorganisms to other patients and environments. Ensure that reusable equipment is not used for the care of another patient until it has been appropriately cleaned and reprocessed and single use items are properly discarded.

Environmental Control
Follow hospital procedures for routine care, cleaning, and disinfection of environmental surfaces, beds, bedrails, bedside equipment and other frequently touched surfaces.

Linen
Handle, transport, and process used linen soiled with blood, body fluids, secretions, or excretions in a manner that prevents exposure and contamination of clothing, and avoids transfer of microorganisms to other patients and environments.

Occupational Health and Bloodborne Pathogens
Prevent injuries when using needles, scalpels, and other sharp instruments or devices; when handling sharp instruments after procedures; when cleaning used instruments; and when disposing of used needles.

Never recap used needles using both hands or any other technique that involves directing the point of a needle towards any part of the body; rather, use either a one-handed "scoop" technique or a mechanical device designed for holding the needle sheath.

Do not remove used needles from disposable syringes by hand, and do not bend, break, or otherwise manipulate used needles by hand. Place used disposable syringes and needles, scalpels, blades, and other sharp items in puncture-resistant sharps containers located as close as practical to the area in which the items were used, and place reusable syringes and needles in a puncture-resistant container for transport to the reprocessing area.

Use resuscitation devices as an alternative to mouth-to-mouth resuscitation.

Patient Placement
Use a private room for a patient who contaminates the environment or who does not (or cannot be expected to) assist in maintaining appropriate hygiene or environmental control. Consult Infection Control if a private room is not available.

Figure 9–9 Standard precautions (Courtesy of BREVIS Corporation, Salt Lake City, UT).

Personal Protective Equipment

personal protective equipment (PPE) provides a barrier between the client and the health care worker and prevents the transfer of pathogens from one person to another

Personal protective equipment (PPE) provides a barrier between the client and the health care worker. When used correctly, PPE provides a barrier that prevents the transfer of pathogens from one person to another. Standard precautions require all health care workers to wear PPE any time they expect to have contact with:

- blood
- moist body fluids except sweat, secretions, or excretions
- mucous membranes
- nonintact skin

PPE includes gloves, water-resistant gowns, face shields, and masks and goggles. HCAs should follow their agency's policies for use of PPE in routine tasks.

Some new medical terms associated with infection control include:

Visible—able to be seen with the eye

Body Substance Isolation—precautions that require special handling of all fluids

Drug Resistant—disease-causing organisms that resist treatment with normal antibiotics

Reservoir—a human being who has an infection that can be spread to others.

Airborne Transmission—disease is spread in the air over long distances such as with TB.

Contact Transmission—disease is spread through direct contact with body fluids such as with HIV.

Droplet Transmission—disease is spread by respiratory secretions or droplets in the air within a distance of three feet.

Transmission-Based Precautions—CDC recommendations for isolating clients with certain diseases in addition to those listed in the standard precautions (see Table 9–1).

Table 9–1 Diseases Requiring Transmission-Based Isolation Precautions	
Disease or Condition	**Type of Precautions**
AIDS	Standard (or reverse if facility policy)
Chickenpox	Airborne and Contact
Diarrhea	Standard
Drug Resistant Skin Infections	Contact
German Measles	Droplet
Head or Body Lice	Contact
Hepatitis, Type A	Standard. Use contact if diarrhea or incontinent patient.
Hepatitis, Other Types	Standard
HIV Disease	Standard
Impetigo	Contact
Infected Pressure Sore with no Drainage	Standard
Infected Pressure Sore with Heavy Drainage	Contact
Infectious Diarrhea Caused by a Known Pathogen	Contact
Measles	Airborne
Mumps	Droplet
Oral or Genital Herpes	Standard
Scabies	Contact
Syphilis	Standard
Tuberculosis of the Lungs	Airborne
Widespread Shingles	Airborne and Contact
Use standard precautions in addition to other types of precautions listed.	

Higher-Efficiency Particulate Air Mask (HEPA)—a special mask with tiny pores to prevent airborne transmission of disease.

Pathogens, which are the cause of infections, can be controlled with good cleaning techniques and maintenance. It is important to keep an **aseptic** environment for the client. The following are some common aseptic practices:

aseptic   absence of pathogens

- Wash hands before and after touching the client.
- Wash hands after urinating, having a bowel movement, or changing tampons or sanitary napkins.
- Wash hands before handling or preparing food.
- Wash fruits and vegetables before serving them.
- Encourage each family member to use his or her own towels, washcloths, toothbrush, drinking glass, and other personal care items.
- Use disposable cups and dishes for clients with an infection.
- Encourage the client to cover the nose and mouth with tissues when coughing, sneezing, or blowing the nose. Make sure there is a plastic or paper bag for used tissues.
- Practice good personal hygiene. Bathe, wash hair, and brush teeth regularly.
- Encourage clients to wash their hands often. They should wash their hands after toileting and before eating.
- Wash cooking and eating utensils with soap and water after they have been used.
- Clean cooking and eating surfaces with soap and water or a disinfectant.
- Do not leave food sitting out and uncovered. Close all food containers. Refrigerate foods that could spoil.
- Do not use food that smells bad or looks discolored.
- Check the expiration date on food. Do not use it if the date has passed.
- Change water in flower vases daily.
- Remove dead plants and flowers from the home.
- Dust furniture with a damp cloth and use a damp mop on floors. This helps prevent the movement of dust in the air.
- Empty garbage every day. Use large, sturdy plastic bags or wrap the garbage in several thicknesses of newspaper. Place the garbage outside the home. If possible, put the bags in plastic or metal garbage containers.
- Wear disposable gloves if there are open cuts or sores on hands.
- Hold equipment and linens away from uniform.

- Do not shake linens. Not shaking helps prevent the movement of dust.
- Clean from the cleanest area to the dirtiest. This prevents soiling a clean area.
- Clean away from the body and uniform. Dusting, brushing, or wiping toward oneself transmits microorganisms to the skin, hair, and uniform.
- Pour contaminated liquids directly into sinks or toilets. Avoid splashing the liquid onto other areas.
- Do not sit on the client's bed if the client has an infection to prevent picking up microorganisms and carrying them to the next surface.
- Wear disposable gloves during contact with the client's body fluids. This includes giving enemas, cleaning the client's genital area, handling vomitus, and giving mouth care.
- Wear a disposable apron when in contact with the client's body fluids.

REVIEW QUESTIONS

1. A safe environment is defined as:

2. List two sensory disabilities that affect the elderly client's safety.
   a.
   b.
3. List the five rights for safety in taking medications.
   a.
   b.
   c.
   d.
   e.
4. Who does the Admission Safety Assessment of the client and the home?
   a. physician
   b. risk manager
   c. nurse
   d. HCA

5. Which of the following are common safety hazards?
   a. wet floors
   b. damaged wiring
   c. poisons
   d. cluttered hallways
   e. all of the above

6. Which of the following is *not* an HCA responsibility?
   a. safe storage of medications
   b. administering medications
   c. assisting the client with medications
   d. measuring medications

7. True or False? If more than one person in a household is taking medications, the medications should be placed in separate rooms.

8. True or False? Old medications should not be flushed down the toilet.

9. True or False? The HCA should know his or her limitations in emergency situations.

10. True or False? It is never acceptable to cover the client's face with a damp cloth when escaping a smoke-filled room.

11. True or False? The CDC has developed new universal precautions entitled standard precautions.

12. True or False? The HCA can lower the risk of transmission of pathogens by using proper hand-washing procedures.

13. Unscramble the following key term from the chapter: ghtnoeap _____

Abuse

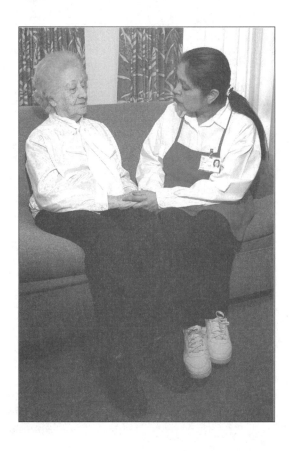

OBJECTIVES

Upon reading this chapter and completing the review questions, the home care aide should be able to:

1. Define the term abuse.
2. Identify six types of abuse and/or neglect.
3. Identify factors contributing to adult abuse.
4. Identify physical indicators of adult abuse, neglect, and exploitation.

KEY TERMS

abuse	intervention
exploitation	self-abuse

INTRODUCTION

abuse inflicting physical or mental pain or injury on another person

Many elderly persons live rich and productive lives with positive relationships with their children and friends. Others are severely disabled and live in institutions. Twice as many live with, and are dependent on, their children or siblings. Those elderly persons who are dependent are often a physical, financial, and emotional strain on those persons and families who care for them. Caring for a dependent older adult in the home can cost up to twenty-five thousand dollars a year. Furthermore, custodial care is not a Medicare reimbursable service and is rarely covered by other health insurance policies. With these two factors common in our society, the 1990s have seen an increase in the neglect and **abuse** of the elderly population.

Abuse is defined as the infliction of physical pain or injury or any persistent course of conduct intended to produce or result in mental or emotional distress. Severe neglect and severe physical abuse cause great distress and pain and can lead to injury or death.

Clients not fully able to care for themselves are easy targets for abuse. This abuse can be administered by untrained, frustrated, or overburdened family members or by those who deliberately harm others for their own gain.

SIX TYPES OF ABUSE

HCAs are in a position to notice signs of abuse or neglect. If either is occurring, whatever is seen should be handled confidentially. Any signs or abuse or suspicions should be reported to the supervisor immediately. The six types of abuse or neglect to watch for are:

1. Passive Neglect—Harm is not intended but occurs because some type of care is not being provided as a result of the caregiver's inability, laziness, or lack of knowledge.

2. Psychological Abuse—Harm is caused to the client's feelings or emotional state by means of the client being demeaned, frightened, humiliated, intimidated, isolated, insulted, or by being treated as a child or as a victim of verbal aggression.

exploitation to use selfishly or unethically

3. Material or Financial Abuse.—Stealing, **exploitation**, or improper use of the money, property, or other assets of the elderly client.

4. Active Neglect—Intentional harm of the older person, physically or psychologically, by failing to provide needed care. Examples include deliberately leaving a bedridden person alone for lengthy periods of time or willfully denying the person food, medication, fluids, dentures, or eyeglasses.

self-abuse infliction of physical or mental injury upon oneself or refusing care necessary for life

5. Physical Abuse—Intentional physical harm of the person by such actions as slapping, bruising, sexually molesting, cutting, burning, physically restraining, pushing, or shoving.

6. **Self-Abuse** or Self-Neglect—Any of the activities mentioned above committed by the older person to himself or herself.

The key for the HCA is to be alert to the physical and mental condition of the client at all times, and to report changes and unusual conditions to the supervisor regularly and promptly.

REPORTING ABUSE

Helpful Hints: The law requires that domestic violence and elder and child abuse be reported by all health caregivers.

Supervisors must be informed of any suspicions the HCA has in order to help identify the proper action to be taken regarding the reporting of abusive behavior. In order to protect the victim, the situation must be handled carefully; the supervisor and other professionals will become involved if it appears that abuse is taking place.

Primary reasons for not reporting elder abuse are:

- fear of personal involvement
- lack of evidence that abuse has occurred
- lack of response by authorities
- a generalized belief that reported cases are not satisfactorily handled

There is a responsibility of health care providers to report discovered cases of abuse, neglect, or exploitation and forty-one states have laws that mandate the reporting of elder abuse. The law usually states that health professionals or persons who have knowledge of abuse or who reasonably suspect abuse must report it. These states also protect the health care personnel from civil or criminal liability for the content of the report. Penalties are issued in some states for not reporting abuse.

FACTORS CONTRIBUTING TO ELDER ABUSE

The factors contributing to elder abuse include:

- retaliation
- ageism (discrimination against the elderly) and violence as a way of life
- lack of close family ties
- lack of community resources
- lack of financial resources
- mental and emotional disorders
- unemployment

- history of alcohol and/or drug abuse
- environmental conditions
- resentment of dependency
- increased life expectancy
- other situational stresses

SIGNS OF ELDER ABUSE

The three main indicators of elder abuse are:

1. Personal factors such as ignorance and emotional disturbance.
2. Interpersonal factors such as unresolved conflicts and lack of gratitude.
3. Situational factors such as dependent persons living with their children and their families, thereby creating feelings of frustration and stress in the caregiver.

   Physical signs of elder abuse, neglect, or exploitation include:

- unexplained bruises or welts
- unexplained fractures
- unexplained burns
- unexplained lacerations or abrasions
- confusion
- poor personal hygiene
- denial of pain
- bedbound but unrelated to the disease
- weight loss
- dehydration
- old, unexplained scars
- fearfulness and noncommunicative

   Behavioral signs of abuse occur when the client:

- yells obscenities at others
- threatens self-harm or suicide
- refuses medical care
- shows unrealistic fear or hostility
- shows signs of alcohol and/or drug abuse
- experiences denial of the situation
- stops communicating
- is fearful of being alone
- cries excessively
- displays anger at the family

- has a poor self-concept and shows poor self-control
- shows signs of hopelessness
  Environmental signs of elder abuse are evidenced by:
- a dirty house with garbage around
- fleas, mice, or vermin present in the home
- an overcrowded home
- the home smells of urine or feces
- the home is not kept at a comfortable temperature
- pets are not well cared for
- empty bottles of liquor or medicine containers are lying around
- bed sheets are dirty and have not been changed
- lack of food in the home
- food is spoiled and the refrigerator is dirty
- food is stored improperly
- special foods for the client's diet are missing
- no available cash
- unusual withdrawals of money from bank account(s)
- complaints of "no money" or "the family is stealing money" by the client

SUBSTANCE ABUSE IN THE ELDERLY

Substance abuse is a causative factor in elder abuse. Abuse of alcohol is a major health problem and the third most common mental disorder in elderly men is alcoholism. Some signs the HCA should watch for in clients that may indicate alcoholism are:

- poor personal hygiene
- nutritional problems (weight loss)
- neglect of the home
- depression
- suicidal ideas
- repeated falls
- flushed face
- tremors
- extreme fatigue
- incontinence
- withdrawal

HCAs should discuss any suspected substance abuse with the supervisor so that the physician can be notified and orders for **intervention** and referral given. The HCA should have good com-

intervention action taken to make a change

munication with the client in order to determine if substance abuse is occurring (see Figure 10–1).

PREVENTION TECHNIQUES

Some suggestions for patients to prevent abuse and maintain independence are:

- keep a network of friends and activities as long as possible
- participate in community activities
- have a "buddy system" with a friend outside the family and communicate weekly
- make and keep personal care appointments such as a dentist and hairdresser
- invite guests to the home often
- maintain his or her own telephone
- be neat and organized
- do not leave valuables around
- do not give up financial control if at all possible

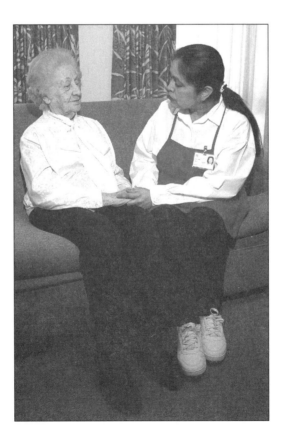

Figure 10–1   HCAs should watch and listen for signs of abuse.

REVIEW QUESTIONS

State the type of abuse described in each of the situations in Questions 1 to 5:

1. A daughter helped her elderly mother by cashing, depositing, and managing all of her income. All purchases and household bills were made for the mother by the daughter using the mother's checkbook. The daughter, unfortunately, also paid her own bills from her mother's account. _____

2. A wife cares for her overweight husband at home after a heart attack. A hospital bed was purchased but the wife was never instructed to turn the patient or give skin care. She and a neighbor discovered, upon turning the husband three weeks later, that he had developed three large bedsores. _____

3. A couple cared for the wife's elderly mother in their home. The patient was very confused and constantly caused disruptions. Her bedroom was cleared and she was locked in day and night. The couple insisted they did the best they could. The mother was moved to a nursing home but the couple refused to pay the bill. _____

4. A daughter asked her elderly mother to move in with her after the daughter's divorce. The daughter began to date and was away many times during the evening hours. The daughter began to resent the mother's verbal concerns and excessive name-calling and threats to the mother ensued. The mother ran away for three days but was returned in a frightened state by the police. _____

5. An alcoholic son lived with his elderly, sick, obese mother in her home. She was hospitalized for fractures of the hip and jaw and bruises on her face and body. The neighbors complained that the son would not allow his mother to leave the house and she died a short time later. Autopsy reports showed that regular beatings had taken place. _____

6. Which of the following are possible signs of abuse in the elderly?
   a. no access to bank accounts
   b pressure sores
   c. poor hygiene
   d. fearfulness
   e. all of the above

7. Behavioral signs of elder abuse include:
   a. bruises and welts
   b. crying and depression
   c. fearfulness
   d. burns

8. True or False? HCAs can make a difference in helping clients maintain independence.

9. True or False? The HCA is required by law to report suspected abuse.

10. True or False? A sign of potential abuse is that garbage is left around the home and the family pets are not well cared for.

11. Unscramble the following key term from the chapter: ronntivieent _____

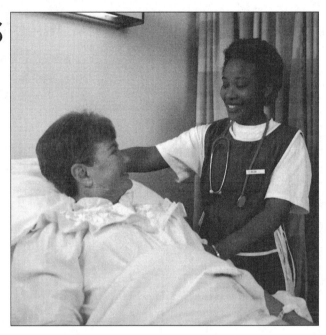

CHAPTER 11

Psychosocial Influences

OBJECTIVES

psychosocial human interaction

Upon reading this chapter and completing the review questions, the home care aide should be able to:

1. Define **psychosocial** influences on the client and his or her recovery.
2. Define holistic care of the client requiring rehabilitation.
3. Understand multicultural differences and human needs.
4. Describe family dynamics and current changes that might affect the client.
5. Be familiar with positive attitudes and codes of HCA behavior.
6. Understand disabilities and human responses to them.
7. Understand the communication process, especially among the elderly and impaired.

KEY TERMS

advocate

confidentiality

cultures

disability

family dynamics

holistic caring model

impairments

psychosocial

INTRODUCTION

Clients receiving home health care live in a family-structured environment. The psycho (emotional) and social (human interactions) influences on the client can affect the rehabilitation process. The HCA should be aware of these influential factors to better provide the client with a more holistic approach to healing.

THE HOLISTIC CARING MODEL

holistic caring model   physical and emotional care based on the belief that humans should be cared for as a "whole" person

advocate   someone who supports and encourages another person

The **holistic caring model** considers the whole client which includes mind, body, spiritual well-being, economy, family support, culture, and ethics. It is important to look at the illness or disease process to see how these other factors affect the recovery of the client.

The HCA serves as a client **advocate** (supporter), but he or she cannot be successful without an understanding of the uniqueness and variety of types of clients and families with needs that require special care and concern. Figure 11–1 shows the HCA as the client's key supporter.

The United States has a growing elderly population as well as an increasing multicultural and multiethnic mix. The HCA of the 1990s will be placed in the homes of persons with differences that could affect the level of care or create barriers to the relationship. Some of the barriers the HCA might see in the home include:

- language differences
- discrimination and distrust

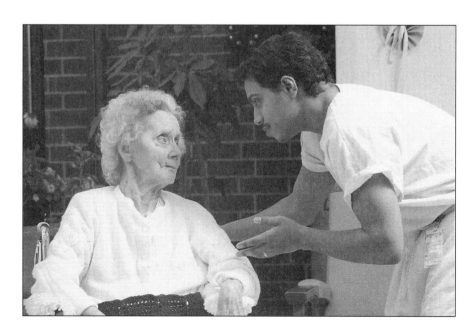

Figure 11–1   The HCA is the client's key supporter.

Helpful Hints: If caregivers believe there is a cultural barrier between them and their client or the family, they should discuss a change of assignment with the supervisor.

- poverty
- resistance to outside help
- culture bias
- negative attitude toward Western health care
- religious practices
- lack of knowledge of the medical system
- lack of education
- misunderstood family structure

Multicultural differences can occur in race, religion, language, dietary habits, gender, age, economic status, and lifestyle.

The one area all human beings have in common is **basic needs**. Certain needs must be met for a person's well-being. The health caregiver should focus on the client/family's needs first, then assess the differences and merge the two to create a care plan for each individual situation. All humans have needs which can be divided into daily physical needs and daily psychological needs.

Daily physical needs:

- food and water
- safety and shelter
- activity and rest
- freedom from pain and discomfort

Daily psychological needs:

- independence and security
- affection and love
- acceptance and social interaction (see Figure 11–2)

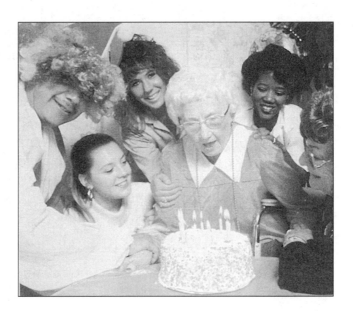

Figure 11–2 Socialization and activities are important components of rehabilitative care.

- trust and dignity
- self-esteem and relationships
- knowledge and achievement

FAMILY DYNAMICS

The family as a unit has changed over the past few decades. The primary family—formerly mother, father, and children—is now frequently made up of step-parents, step-children, and half-brothers and half-sisters. The extended family—grandparents, aunts, and uncles—who used to live in the same location, are now scattered over large geographical areas. As travel became easier, families moved to separate parts of the country. Changes in the family unit are the result of many factors such as:

- smaller families
- single-parent families
- divorces and second marriages
- interracial families
- two-career families
- same-sex households
- aging elderly
- baby boomers
- multicultural families
- diversity and blending of ethnic groups

family dynamics how the family interacts with each other

The **family dynamics** in the home also have been greatly influenced. Factors contributing to differences in the family that might affect the client include:

- increase in medical technology
- growth of new minority groups
- blend of cultures in diet, religion, and customs
- differences in health practices and beliefs
- family structure
- language and communication barriers

All these factors and differences that influence the client and the family's behavior and acceptance of them by the health care members is the key to understanding. If, however, the HCA believes the behavior in some way interferes with the client's recovery, it is important to report it to the supervisor.

COMMUNICATION

Of all the factors affecting relationships and interactions between client/family and the HCA, communication is so important that it

impairments injury or dysfunction

requires further discussion. The United States is a melting pot of many cultures with many different languages and various methods of communication. In addition, the client in a rehabilitation program may be elderly, with hearing, speaking, and visual **impairments**, that can create even more problems in the communication process.

Proper communication is not only what is said but also the way in which it is expressed. Gestures and facial expressions are also important elements of communication. A positive and cheerful attitude, which is also professional, promotes a trusting relationship between HCA and client (see Figure 11–3)

Some general guidelines to improve communication skills include:

- a calm and supportive attitude
- touch, and a caring behavior when reassuring the client (see Figure 11-4)
- eye contact
- slow and distinctive speech delivered in a lower pitch and tone
- one question asked at a time with plenty of time allowed for a response

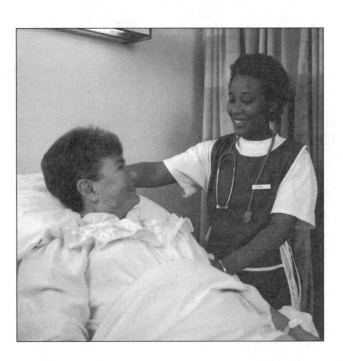

Figure 11–3 A positive and cheerful attitude promotes a trusting relationship between the HCA and the client.

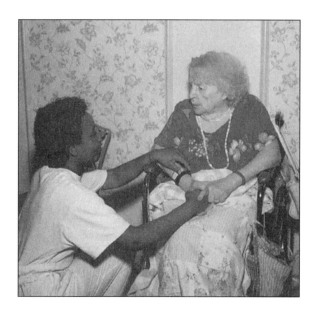

Figure 11–4 Touch and a caring behavior reassure the client.

- communication that shows respect and dignity to the client, especially the elderly and disabled
- articulate speech when conversing with friends and family; each word must be spoken clearly, especially when speaking to someone who is hard of hearing or whose native language is not English
- patience, and learning to listen until the message is completed by the sender, even if the sender has a difficult time stating the message (time spent here is time saved later)
- using agreed-upon modes of communication when speaking to clients or families who speak languages or come from cultures other than those of the HCA/caregiver
- do not use words or phrases from another language you do not understand unless taught to you by the client or family

Communicating with the elderly is vital in gaining information important to the nurse and/or physician. The HCA must remember that the elderly think and speak more slowly than other clients and must not be rushed. Noise and distractions should be kept to a minimum and short, simple words and sentences used. The nurse will determine if the client has impairments such as hearing, seeing, or speaking.

Helpful Hints: HCAs should keep well informed about each client's impairments so that special considerations can be determined.

Hearing Impairments

The hearing impaired present a special situation for the HCA. The following communication techniques have been broken down into supportive (those that improve the communication process) and nonsupportive (those techniques that make the situation worse) in working with clients who have hearing impairments.

Supportive communication techniques:

1. Speak clearly, slowly, in good lighting, and directly facing the hearing impaired client (see Figure 11–5).

2. Be sure to get the client's attention before speaking. Do not start to speak abruptly.

3. Lower the tone of your voice. Telephone bells, doorbells, horns, and emergency alarms should be toned down also.

4. Repeat what is said, using different words, whenever necessary.

5. Know in which ear the client has better hearing and speak to that side.

6. Recognize that hearing decline is a normal aspect of aging. Convey this understanding through a supportive attitude.

7. Help family members or those who work with older clients become better speakers by pointing out helpful speech habits such as those listed above.

Nonsupportive communication techniques:

1. Shouting increases nonintelligible sounds and grossly distorts what the client hears.

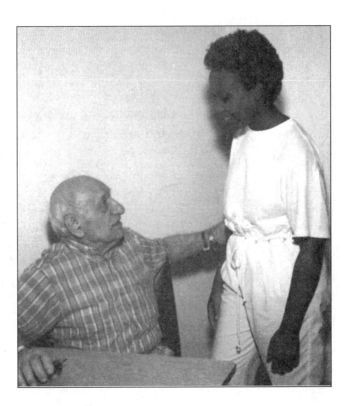

Figure 11–5 Face the hearing-impaired client directly and speak slowly and distinctly.

2. Background noise, such as traffic or many persons talking at once.

3. Speaking too softly, running words together, or looking away from the hearing-impaired client while speaking.

4. Nonsupportive behaviors that interfere with lip reading. These include:

   • exaggerated or distorted speech movements by persons trying to help the lip reader

   • speech that is too rapid

   • poor lighting on the speaker's face

   • mustaches that cover the lip

   • anything that covers the speaker's mouth such as cigars, pencils, fingers, food, or gum

Visual Impairments

Working with clients who have visual impairments is another special situation that requires good communication techniques geared to that particular situation. The following are some guidelines:

1. If the client has eyeglasses, make sure they are clean and that he or she wears them. Also, make sure that glasses are in good repair and fit correctly.

2. Provide adequate lighting at all times. Pools of bright light among darkened areas or variations in light intensity should be avoided.

3. Reduce glare by avoiding shiny surfaces, waxed floors, and exposed light bulbs. Have shades or sheer curtains at windows to reduce glare.

4. Use dishes with brightly colored rims to reduce spills.

5. Use sharply contrasting colors for doors, bedspreads, floors, and walls to help clients find their way and reduce accidents.

6. Provide large print newspapers, magazines, and books.

7. Refer to positions on the face of a clock to help the client locate items on a dinner plate or tray.

8. Ensure that clients with decreased peripheral vision are aware of people or items sitting beside them.

9. Provide black telephones with white numerals because they are easier to see.

10. Do not move personal belongings or rearrange furniture without the client's knowledge.

11. Consistently use sensory stimulations of sound, touch, and smell.

12. Use large clocks, clocks that chime, and radios to keep the client oriented to time.

13. Obtain "talking books" and other low-vision aids.

14. Ensure that numerals on doors and dials (such as a stove) are large and distinct enough for clients with visual impairments to see or feel.

15. Use magnifying glasses as a visual aid whenever necessary.

16. Give simple instructions and explanations for anything you plan to do such as moving the client.

17. Use sunglasses, sun visors, caps, or hats with brims to help with glare on rainy days or when there is snow on the ground.

Speaking Impairments (Aphasia)

Communicating with clients who have difficulty speaking (aphasia) creates another health care challenge. Clients who have had strokes are slow to regain their speaking abilities and require increased patience on the part of the HCA. Some important principles to remember in this situation include:

1. Reduce your rate of speaking by prolonging the pauses between words and phrases when helping a client who is learning to speak.

2. Speak in a normal tone of voice, emphasize the main ideas, and use gestures to help clarify meanings.

3. Ask questions that can be answered with "yes" or "no" when requiring reliable information. For example, if the HCA wants to know what the client drank at dinner, ask "Did you have milk?" instead of "Did you have milk, coffee, or tea?"

4. Do not supply an anticipated word unless the client requests it because aphasia frequently causes a client frustration and embarrassment.

5. Do not talk about a client in his or her presence. It is rude and can be discouraging to the client. Aphasic clients, especially, may understand but be unable to express their thoughts and feelings.

6. Be accepting of errors and understand that speech and language will improve with time and proper training.

7. Never speak to adult clients as though they were children. Doing so creates hurt feelings that could lead to frustration and depression, or feelings of resentment against the speaker. Adult clients, regardless of their abilities, are not children and do not deserve to be treated as such.

8. Do not attempt to continue tasks that are frustrating to the client for long periods of time. Aphasic clients have a reduced ability to attend to activities for long periods of time and tire quickly. Arrange for short periods of activity and seek improvements in small steps so that some successes are achieved at each session.

9. Discourage clients from remaining alone all day. When possible, provide clients with opportunities for interacting with others in order for them to see that they are accepted and can enjoy life despite their aphasic difficulties.

10. Write down what is to be conveyed if the accuracy of a message is critical, or if reinforcement of verbal and nonverbal communication is desired.

11. Give positive reinforcement—both verbal and nonverbal—of the client's progress.

The ultimate goal in communication with home care clients is to provide the best ongoing care possible. Sometimes this means making changes in care based on the information the HCA sees and hears. If a supervisor deems the changes serious enough, he or she will speak to the doctor to determine if the orders should be reevaluated.

Helpful Hints: Clients with hearing, visual, or speech impairments tend to avoid interaction with others. HCAs should encourage them to overcome these barriers.

STRESSES ON THE ELDERLY CLIENT

Factors that cause stress to the elderly client and influence his or her recovery that the HCA should be aware of include:

- disturbance in sleep patterns
- loss of friends
- loneliness
- fear of illness
- loss of a beloved pet
- decreasing eyesight
- decreasing hearing
- loss of mental abilities
- fear of impending death
- economic losses and concerns
- loss of driver's license
- fear of hospitalization
- illness of a significant other
- feelings of dependency
- wish for more family visits
- less ability to care for oneself

- death of family member or close friend
- use of assistive devices
- loss of prior social or recreational activities
- regrets
- missing children

CONFIDENTIALITY

confidentiality not taking the client's personal information outside the workplace

Confidentiality means that information about the client/family is personal and should not be repeated to persons outside of the workplace. The HCA must follow the basic guidelines for confidentiality:

- discuss the client's medical and personal facts only with the health care team
- it is the physician's responsibility to tell the client medical information
- do not discuss co-workers or workplace problems with peers or family; go directly to the supervisor (see Figure 11–6).

Helpful Hints: Clients in nursing homes or assisted care living facilities are very curious about other clients and their private lives. Be courteous but do not give personal information concerning one client to another.

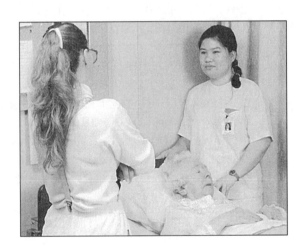

Figure 11–6 HCAs should not discuss personal activities in the presence of the client or family.

HCA BEHAVIORS AND ATTITUDES

culture behavior patterns or lifestyles of a particular race, nation, or group of people

HCAs come from many **cultures** and backgrounds. Each HCA brings his or her ethics or code of behavior to the home which is his or her workplace. These include:

- honesty with peers and clients
- respect of the client's home
- acceptance of differences in families
- reporting abuse
- caring for yourself and your appearance

- knowing and respecting the client's rights
- keeping a cheerful and positive attitude
- being dependable and on time
- never leaving the workplace with work unfinished
- never accepting tips or gifts
- knowing the HCA's rights

Positive attitudes that reflect HCAs of the highest level include:

- being cheerful at tasks
- smiling during visits
- being happy to do "extras"
- having pride in their appearance
- following directions well
- being empathetic to the client
- praising even small client participation
- leaving personal problems at home

disability a permanent condition that causes physical or mental handicaps or weakness

Clients with disabilities are often involved in rehabilitation. These persons require an extra measure of consideration and care. A **disability** is a permanent condition that causes a physical or mental handicap or weakness caused by an accident, birth problem, or illness. Family responses to disabilities vary depending on the dynamics previously discussed. Client responses to disabilities also vary depending on that person's age, psychosocial background, degree of the disability, economic factors, family involvement and attitude, and the client's needs level. Some negative responses the HCA should recognize of client/family to disabilities are anger, denial, silence, and abuse.

All persons with disabilities should be given the opportunities to live at the highest level of self-care and self-respect and in a safe and healthy environment.

REVIEW QUESTIONS

1. List four barriers to the relationship between the HCA and the client/family.
   a.
   b.
   c.
   d.

2. Multicultural differences may occur in which area(s)?

   a. race

   b. religion

   c. language

   d. diet

   e. all of the above

3. Examples of human physical needs are all but which of the following?

   a. food

   b. water

   c. love

   d. rest

4. Which is not a psychological need?

   a. safety

   b. affection

   c. trust

   d. dignity

5. Which of the following are examples of factors contributing to differences in families that may affect the client?

   a. language

   b. technology

   c. cultures

   d. baby boomers

6. True or False? The HCA's acceptance of differences is important for a relationship with the client.

7. True or False? The HCA may discuss medical information with the family.

8. True or False? Anger is a typical client response to a disability.

9. True or False? Decreasing numbers of friends is a source of stress for the elderly client.

10. True or False? The elderly do not feel stressed or concerned about increasing dependency on others.

11. True or False? Touch can be an effective means of communication.

12. True or False? If the client or family wish to teach the HCA some cultural phrases, he or she should refuse.

13. Unscramble the following key term from the chapter: mipienmatr _____

Glossary

abduction   to draw away from the median plane of the body

abrasion   an injury resulting from scraping away a portion of skin or of a mucous membrane

abuse   inflicting physical or mental pain or injury on another person

activities of daily living (ADLs)   tasks performed each day such as toileting, bathing, dressing, feeding, grooming, homemaking, and other activities

adaptive equipment   assists the client with ADLs

adduction   to draw toward the midline of the body

ADL sheet   a written form devised to document the degree of activities of daily living performed at each home visit

advocate   someone who supports and encourages another person

amputation   the surgical removal of all or part of a limb, usually one of the lower extremities, above or below the knee

aphasia   loss of language or speech

arteriosclerosis   a build-up of cholesterol in the arteries

arthritis   an inflammation of the joint causing pain and limitation of movement of the joint

aseptic   absence of pathogens

atrophy   muscle decreasing in size

autonomic nervous system   the involuntary nervous system which controls the function of smooth muscle tissue, the heart, and glands

bladder training   training to restore the client's ability to control urination

body mechanics   correct and safe use of the body for work

bone marrow   the medulla or soft tissues in the hollow of long bones concerned with production, maintenance, and disposal of red blood cells (RBCs) and hemoglobin

bowel training   training to restore the client's ability to control bowel movements

burnout   exhaustion of one's physical and/or emotional endurance

bursitis   inflammation of the serous sac of a joint such as the elbow or shoulder

care plan   the written plan for daily care and treatments for the client that all disciplines follow

case conference   meetings of all members of the health care team to analyze the client's case

cataracts   a cloudiness of the lens of the eye which obstructs vision

catheter   a flexible tube inserted into the body to drain fluids out or inject fluids

Centers for Disease Control and Prevention (CDC)   an agency of the U.S. Department of Health and Human Services, concerned with all phases of control of communicable and occupational diseases and with prevention of disease, injury, and disability

client information sheet   a form devised to document important information regarding the client, family, and environment

compliance   how well the client/family responds to the educational process

confidentiality   not taking the client's personal information outside the workplace

confused   mentally uncertain or unclear

contracture   when muscle tissue becomes drawn together or shortened because of spasm or paralysis (can be permanent or temporary)

culture   behavior patterns or lifestyles of a particular race, nation, or group of people

cerebral vascular accident (CVA; also called a stroke) a disorder in which blood flow to parts of the brain are blocked caused by a hemorrhage, a thrombus, an embolus, or arteriosclerosis

daily visit form a written form devised to document treatments performed at time of home visit; often vital information for financial reimbursement purposes

decubitus ulcers skin breakdown over body areas due to pressure or friction

diabetic retinopathy a disease of the eye found in some persons with Diabetes Mellitus, characterized by vitreous hemorrhage resulting in possible retinal detachment

disability a permanent condition that causes physical or mental handicaps or weakness

disoriented confusion as to identity or location

distractions activities or techniques to change the client's focus from his or her pain

documentation the written account of care given to a client

edema a condition of body tissue containing grossly abnormal amounts of fluid

education plan the day-to-day organization and process of the client/family teaching procedure prepared by the nurse

elimination the process of urinating

embolus foreign matter which enters the blood stream and obstructs a blood vessel

emesis the act of vomiting

empower to authorize or strongly encourage another person

exercise equipment equipment to improve the strength and mobility of the client

expected outcomes the hoped-for results of short- and long-term goals

exploitation to use selfishly or unethically

extension a movement which brings the parts of a limb into or toward a straight position

family dynamics how the family interacts with each other

flammable able to catch fire

flatus   gas or air in the gastrointestinal tract that, if not expelled through the anus, causes abdominal distension and discomfort

flexion   the act of bending; a condition of being bent

Fowler's position   the patient is in a semi-sitting position with the head of the bed elevated approximately 45 degrees and the mattress or pillows gathered to elevate the knees slightly

fracture   a sudden breaking of a bone

functional limitations   the client's level of ambulation and activity

gait belt   a belt or harness placed around the client's waist to assist with the stabilization of the client when ambulating

gait training   teaching the client the proper gait (walk) with assistive devices

glaucoma   a disease of the eye marked by increased pressure within the eyeball resulting in damage to the retina and gradual loss of vision

goal   purpose or objective to work toward

HCA care plan   plan the HCA follows which is created by the nurse and updated every two weeks

hemorrhage   a large discharge of blood from the blood vessels

hip disorders   disease or injury to the hip such as arthritis, fractures, dislocation, and hip surgery

home maintenance   keeping the home as a safe and healthy environment

holistic caring model   physical and emotional care based on the belief that humans should be cared for as a "whole" person

hypertension   high blood pressure

hypotension   low blood pressure

impairment   injury or dysfunction

incontinence   the inability to control bladder or bowel function

infection   germs entering the body and causing disease

intervention   action taken to make a change

involuntary muscles   muscles that receive messages from the nervous system but work automatically without the person being aware of it

lateral (side-laying) position the patient is positioned on left side, the right thigh and knee drawn up. The opposite is true for right side lateral position.

medical social worker (MSW) deals with spiritual, economic, and psychosocial problems

motivation to encourage another person to action

multidiscipline the group of various therapies (disciplines) on the rehabilitation team

Muscular Dystrophy (MD) a progressive disease characterized by weakness and atrophy of the muscles

myelin sheath a fat-like white material forming a covering of a nerve fiber

Multiple Sclerosis (MS) a central nervous system disease of unknown cause with associated symptoms of weakness, uncoordination, speech disturbances, and visual complaints; the course of the disease is usually prolonged

nerve cell the essential component of nervous tissue; a neuron

nursing care plan plan the nurse follows which consists of problems (nursing diagnoses) and the long- and short-term goals to meet those problems

occupation how the client is occupied in day-to-day living activities

occupational therapist (OT) assists in restoring muscle coordination and strength by increasing the client's activity and independence

osteoarthritis a noninflammatory degenerative joint disease occurring chiefly in older persons

osteoporosis a reduction in the amount of bone mass leading to fractures after minimal trauma

pain management pain control through techniques to reduce discomfort

paraplegic a client whose lower part of the body is paralyzed

Parkinson's disease a chronic nervous system disease characterized by tremors, muscular rigidity, weakness, and decreased mobility

pathogen disease-causing microorganism

payors of home care   Medicare, HMOs, or any insurance company that covers the client's health care expenses

personal care devices   special equipment designed to encourage self-care

personal protective equipment (PPE)   provides a barrier between the client and the health care worker and prevents the transfer of pathogens from one person to another.

phantom pain   the sensation following the amputation of a limb that is still present with pain perceived as originating in the absent limb

physical therapist (PT)   uses exercises and treatments to increase mobility

plantar flexion   contraction of toes upon irritation of the sole of the foot

position change record   a written document to verify when the change of position of bedridden clients was performed by health care personnel

prone   patient lying on abdomen with face to the side and toes over edge of mattress or elevated from bed with pillow

prosthesis   an artificial substitute for a missing body part used for functional or cosmetic reasons, or both

psychosocial   human interaction

PT plan of care   care plan specific to PT care and treatments

quadriplegic   a client in whom all four extremities are paralyzed

range of motion (ROM)   exercises which move each muscle and joint through a full range of motion to assist the patient in an exercise program

rehabilitation center   outpatient PT when large equipment is needed

rehabilitation equipment   helps the client recover or improve activity

respiratory therapist (RT)   restores the best level of breathing through breathing exercises

retention catheter (Foley®)   an indwelling catheter retained in the bladder by means of a balloon inflated with air or liquid and used to drain urine

rheumatoid arthritis   a form of arthritis with inflammation, stiffness, swelling, and pain of the joints

safe environment an environment in which a person has a very low risk of illness or injury

safety devices equipment used to lower the risk of client injury

self-abuse infliction of physical or mental injury upon oneself or refusing care necessary for life

shearing an action or stress caused by applied forces that cause two parts of the body to rub against each other

signs client changes that can be seen, felt, heard, or smelled

spasm an involuntary movement of muscle

speech therapist (ST) assists to improve speech and communication abilities

sprain a sudden or severe twisting of a joint with stretching or tearing of ligaments

standard precautions guidelines published by the CDC to prevent the spread of pathogens to health care workers from their clients

strain bodily injury from excessive tension or exertion

supine patient positioned flat on back with face upward and arms straight at sides

supportive devices protect the client from falling when ambulating

symptoms client's stated complaints

synovial fluid a colorless lubricating fluid of joints, bursae, and tendon sheaths

tendonitis inflammation of the tendons and tendon muscle attachments

TENS unit electrical stimulation of nerves to reduce pain

thrombus a blood clot obstructing a blood vessel or a cavity of the heart

transient ischemic attack (TIA) a brief attack (lasting from a few minutes to an hour or more) of cerebral dysfunction of vascular origin with no persistent deficit

trochanter roll a rolled towel or pillow positioned under hip or other extremity to support or prevent outer rotation of the extremity

TPRs an abbreviation denoting body temperature, pulse, and respiratory rates

universal precautions   guidelines designed as protection for workers in the health care industry to prevent cross-contamination and further infection to themselves and those in their care

vital signs (VS)   a person's temperature, blood pressure, pulse, and respiratory rates; signs necessary for, or pertaining to, life

voluntary muscles   the movement of the body controlled by the conscious brain

weight-bearing   amount of body weight placed on a hip or leg

Index

Reservoir, 125
Respiratory therapist (RT), 33
Rheumatoid arthritis, 12, 13*f*, 14

S

Safe environment, 114
Safety
    emergency measures in home care,
        118–120
    falls, 115–117
    features for the bath, 116*f*
    fire safety, 120–123
    maintaining a safe environment, 114, 115*f*
    medications, 117–118
Safety devices, 41–42
Self-abuse, 131
Self-neglect, 131
Sensory organs, 7
Sheepskin pads, 82
Signs, 53
Skeletal traction, 16
Skin care, 78–82
    decubitus ulcers, 78–79
    position care record, 81*f*
    pressure points, 80*f*
    pressure sores
        assistive devices to prevent, 81–82
        special care to prevent, 82
    skin breakdown
        common sites of, 79*f*
        prevention of, 80
        stages of, 79
Skin traction, 16
Skull, 8f
Small intestine, 5, 6f
Spasm, 23
Speaking impairments (aphasia), 145–146
Speech therapist (ST), 32
Spinal cord, 7*f*, 8
Spinal injuries, 20–21
Standard precautions, 123, 124*f*
Stomach, 5, 6*f*
Stresses on the elderly client, 146–147
Stroke. *See* Cerebral vascular accident (CVA)

Substance abuse in the elderly, 133–134
Supine position, 66
Supportive devices, 42–43, 44*f*
    for repositioning the client, 72–73
Suppository, rectal, insertion of, 86–87
Symptoms, 53

T

Tendons, 2
TENS unit, 103
TIA, 22
Toes, range of motion exercises for, 64
Toilet seats, raised, 42*f*
Traction, 16
Transient ischemic attack (TIA), 22
Transmission-based precautions, 125, 125*t*
Trochanter roll, 73*f*

U

Universal precautions, 123
Ureters, 5, 6*f*
Urethra, 5, 6*f*
Urinary bladder, 5, 6*f*
Urinary system, 4-5, 6*f*
    disorders of, 17-18, 19*f*

V

Visible, 125
Visual impairments, 144–145
Voluntary muscles, 3

W

Walkers, 44*f*
    assisting to walk with, 76–78
Water crate mattress, 81
Weight-bearing, 104
Wheelchairs, locking devices for, 42*f*
Wrist, range of motion exercises for, 63